ARTHUR S. KEATS LIBRARY
W9-BKP-083
TEXAS HEART INSTITUTE

ADVANCES IN

Cardiac Surgery®

VOLUME 8

ADVANCES IN Cardiac Surgery®

VOLUME 1 THROUGH 4 (OUT OF PRINT)

VOLUME 5

Myocardial Edema: Importance in the Study of Left Ventricular Function, *by Henry M. Spotnitz and Daphne T. Hsu*

Complete Myocardial Revascularization With Arterial Conduit, *by Hendrick B. Barner and Reddy J. Vardhan*

Fetal Cardiac Surgery, *by Frank L. Hanley*

Surgical Management of Pulmonary Atresia With Ventricular Septal Defect and Multiple Aortopulmonary Collaterals, *by Lester C. Permut and Hillel Laks*

Interrupted Aortic Arch, *by Warren W. Bailey*

The Bidirectional Glenn Procedure: Palliation of the Univentricular Heart, *by Richard D. Mainwaring, John J. Lamberti, and Karen Uzark*

Progress in Immunosuppression, *by John Dunning and John Wallwork*

Percutaneous Extracorporeal Membrane Oxygenation, *by Ricardo J. Moreno-Cabral, Walter P. Dembitsky, Robert M. Adamson, and Pat O. Daily*

Application of New Pacemaker and Defibrillator Technology, *by Richard B. Shepard, Andrew E. Epstein, and G. Neal Kay*

Implantable Cardioverter Defibrillator, *by Lynda L. Mickleborough*

Cardiac Xenotransplantation: Insurmountable Barrier or Clinical Reality? *by Robert E. Michler, Jonathan M. Chen, and Eric A. Rose*

VOLUME 6

VOLUME 7

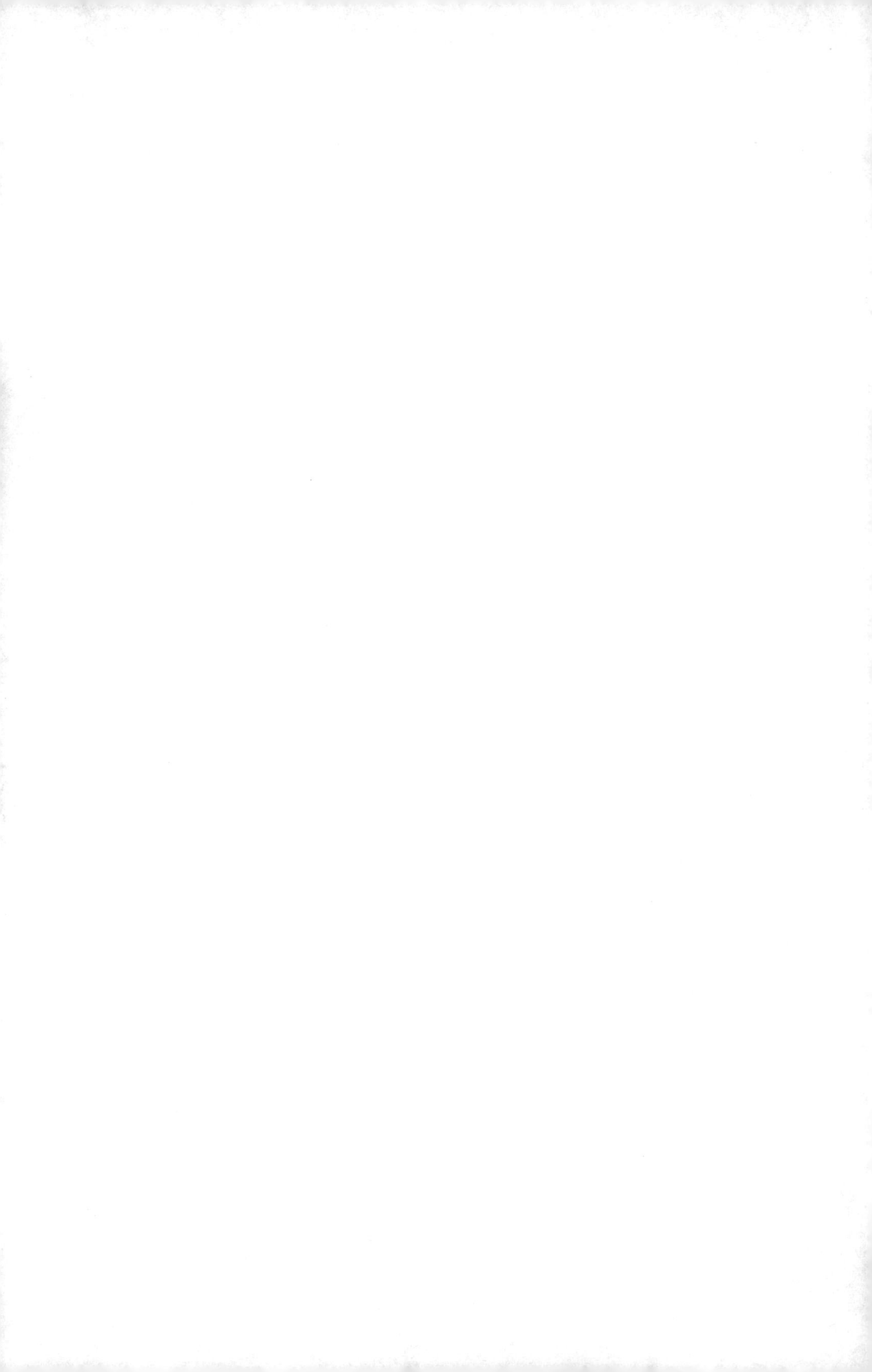

ADVANCES IN Cardiac Surgery®

VOLUME 8

Editor-in-Chief
Robert B. Karp, M.D.
Professor of Surgery, Chief of Cardiac Surgery, University of Chicago, Pritzker School of Medicine, Chicago, Illinois

Editorial Board
Hillel Laks, M.D.
Professor and Chief, Division of Cardiothoracic Surgery; Director, Heart Transplant Program, UCLA Medical Center, Los Angeles, California

Andrew S. Wechsler, M.D.
Stuart McGuire Professor and Chairman, Department of Surgery; Chief, Division of Cardiothoracic Surgery; Professor of Physiology, Medical College of Virginia, Virginia Commonwealth University, Richmond, Virginia

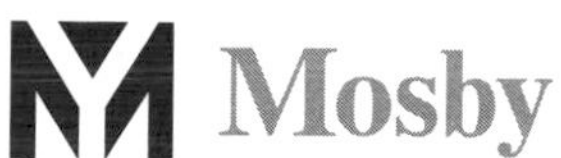

St. Louis Baltimore Boston Carlsbad Chicago Naples New York Philadelphia Portland
London Madrid Mexico City Singapore Sydney Tokyo Toronto Wiesbaden

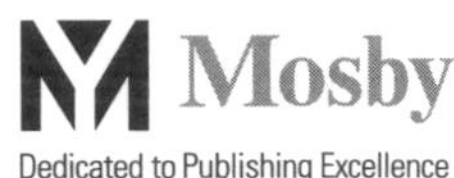

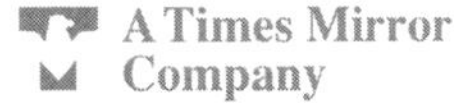

Vice President and Publisher, Continuity Publishing: Kenneth H. Killion
Director, Editorial Development: Gretchen C. Murphy
Acquisitions Editor: Li Wen Huang
Developmental Editor, Continuity: Vivienne F. Heard
Manager, Continuity–EDP: Maria Nevinger
Associate Production Editor: Anna Wleklinski
Assistant Project Supervisor: Sandra Rogers
Freelance Staff Supervisor: Barbara M. Kelly
Circulation Manager: Lynn D. Stevenson

Copyright © 1996 by Mosby–Year Book, Inc.

All rights reserved. No part of this publication may be reproduced, stored in a retrieval system, or transmitted, in any form or by any means, electronic, mechanical, photocopying, recording, or otherwise, without prior written permission from the publisher.

Permission to photocopy or reproduce solely for internal or personal use is permitted for libraries or other users registered with the Copyright Clearance Center, provided that the base fee of $4.00 per chapter plus $.10 per page is paid directly to the Copyright Clearance Center, 27 Congress Street, Salem, MA 01970. This consent does not extend to other kinds of copying, such as copying for general distribution, for advertising or promotional purposes, for creating new collected works, or for resale.

Printed in the United State of America
Composition by The Clarinda Company
Printing/binding by The Maple-Vail Book Manufacturing Group

Mosby–Year Book, Inc.
11830 Westline Industrial Drive
St. Louis, Missouri 63146

Editorial Office:
Mosby–Year Book, Inc.
161 North Clark Street
Chicago, Illinois 60601

International Standard Serial Number: 0889-5074
International Standard Book Number: 0-8151-5099-7

Contributors

Gianni D. Angelini, M.Ch., F.R.C.S.
British Heart Foundation Professor of Cardiac Surgery, Bristol Heart Institute, University of Bristol, Bristol Royal Infirmary, England

Thomas X. Aufiero, M.D.
Associate Professor of Surgery, Indiana University School of Medicine, Indianapolis

Nancy D. Bridges, M.D.
Assistant Professor of Pediatrics (Cardiology), University of Pennsylvania School of Medicine; Medical Director, Lung and Heart/Lung Transplantation and Pulmonary Hypertension Services, Children's Hospital of Philadelphia

John W. Brown, M.D.
Harris B. Shumaker Professor of Surgery and Chief, Section of Cardiovascular Surgery, Indiana University School of Medicine, Indianapolis

Alan J. Bryan, D.M., F.R.C.S.
Senior Lecturer, Bristol Heart Institute, University of Bristol, Bristol Royal Infirmary, England

Richard P. Cochran, M.D.
Associate Professor, Division of Cardiothoracic Surgery, University of Washington, Seattle

Karyn S. Kunzelman, Ph.D.
Research Assistant Professor, Division of Cardiothoracic Surgery; Adjunct Faculty, Center for Bioengineering, University of Washington, Seattle

Luiz Felipe P. Moreira, M.D., Ph.D.
Cardiovascular Surgeon, Heart Institute, São Paulo University Medical School, Brazil

Ivan M. Rebeyka, M.D.
Associate Professor of Surgery and Physiology, University of Toronto; Staff Cardiovascular Surgeon, The Hospital for Sick Children, Toronto

D. Royston, F.R.C.A.
Consultant in Cardiothoracic Anaesthesia, Harefield Hospital, Middlesex, England

Thomas L. Spray, M.D.
Professor of Surgery, University of Pennsylvania School of Medicine; Chief, Cardiothoracic Surgery and Director, Thoracic Organ Transplantation, Children's Hospital of Philadelphia

Noedir A.G. Stolf, M.D., Ph.D.
Associated Professor, Department Cardio-Thoracic Surgery; Cardiovascular Surgeon, Heart Institute, São Paulo University Medical School, Brazil

Kung Sun, M.D., Ph.D.
Korea University Medical Center, Seoul

Contents

Intraoperative Neonatal Myocardial Management: Protection vs. Injury

Ivan M. Rebeyka, M.D.
Associate Professor of Surgery and Physiology, University of Toronto;
Staff Cardiovascular Surgeon, The Hospital for Sick Children, Toronto

The surgical treatment of complex congenital heart defects in the neonate requires controlled conditions with unimpaired exposure in a bloodless, immobile operative field. The cost one pays to obtain such exposure, however, is a period of ischemic insult to the myocardium. Although the importance of minimizing surgically induced myocardial ischemia is obvious, the role of myocardial protection in neonatal cardiac surgery remains controversial among congenital surgeons. Contrasting views are held, not only as to which methods optimally protect the neonatal heart, but also regarding the relative importance of myocardial protection in determining operative results. This diversity in opinion is reflected in the neonatal myocardial protection techniques used in various centers. In 1990, a survey of 127 pediatric cardiac surgery centers in North America revealed an almost equal split in the preference for crystalloid vs. blood cardioplegic solutions.[1] A more recent update of this survey, performed in 1995, indicates a trend toward the use of blood-based solutions, with only 20% of centers currently using crystalloid solutions exclusively.

At present, our incomplete understanding of the fundamental physiologic effects of cardioplegic ischemic arrest in the neonatal heart precludes any claim that one particular method or technique provides optimal myocardial protection in all situations. Undoubtedly, many factors interact in a complex fashion to influence postoperative myocardial function. This chapter addresses several areas of controversy regarding neonatal myocardial protection and highlights potentially harmful factors that may exacerbate myocardial injury in the clinical setting.

© 1996, Mosby–Year Book, Inc.

IS INADEQUATE MYOCARDIAL PROTECTION AN IMPORTANT CAUSE OF POSTOPERATIVE MORBIDITY AND MORTALITY IN NEONATAL CARDIAC SURGERY?

Although some believe that primary myocardial dysfunction in the absence of residual anatomical defects is a rare cause of postoperative death, numerous clinical reports have inferred that inadequate myocardial protection significantly contributes to the morbidity and mortality associated with neonatal cardiac surgery. The report cited most frequently regarding the limitations of cardioplegic protection in pediatric cardiac surgery is that of Bull and associates. On the basis of cytochemical and biophysical assessment of right ventricular biopsy specimens obtained before and after intraoperative ischemia, they demonstrated that hypothermic cardioplegia conferred inadequate protection beyond 85 minutes of ischemia and concluded that the resulting myocardial injury accounted for 50% of perioperative deaths.[2] A subsequent clinical study by Hammon and colleagues found that postischemic myocardial levels of adenosine triphosphate (ATP) were less than 40% of preischemic values in 7 of 20 patients after repair of congenital cardiac lesions. Further, the reduction in ATP levels correlated with depression of ventricular function and low cardiac output postoperatively.[3] Perhaps the best controlled and most convincing clinical study supporting the impression of an altered response to intraoperative myocardial ischemia in immature vs. mature myocardium is the report of Lofland and co-workers. In this study, right ventricular biopsy specimens obtained before and after 45 minutes of surgical ischemia in patients younger than 18 months of age were compared with those of patients older than 18 months. Despite similar myocardial protection techniques in both age groups, there was a highly significant reduction in postischemic ATP levels in the younger age group[4] (Fig 1).

In contrast to these clinical studies suggesting that neonatal myocardium is more susceptible to intraoperative damage in the surgical setting, most experimental studies have concluded that immature myocardium has an inherently greater tolerance to hypoxia and normothermic ischemia.[5–8] The relative increased resistance to ischemia in immature myocardium has been attributed to several factors, including a greater capacity for anaerobic glycolysis, a greater buffering capacity, and decreased ATP efflux secondary to lower levels of 5-nucleotidase. Several reports have suggested that immature myocardium is less tolerant to ischemia based on the duration of ischemia at the onset of contracture or intracellular accumulation of sodium and calcium,[9–11] but recovery of pump function was not assessed.

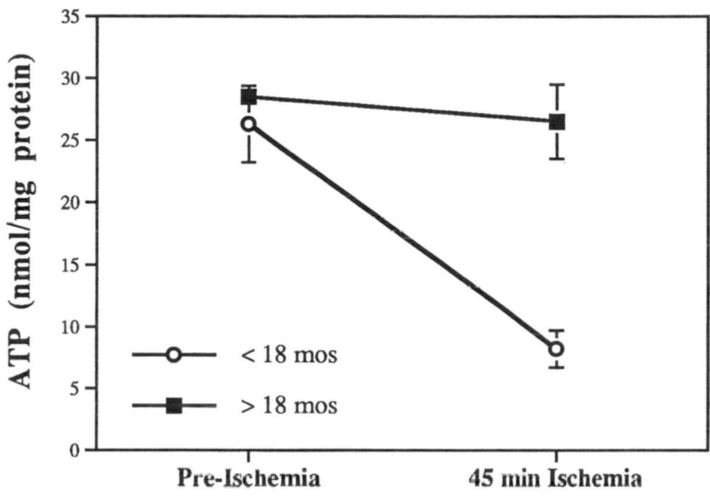

FIGURE 1.
Myocardial levels of adenosine triphosphate (ATP) before and after 45 minutes of cardioplegic arrest in patients younger and older than 18 months of age. (Adapted from Lofland G, Abd-Elfattah A, Wyse R, et al: Myocardial adenine nucleotide metabolism in pediatric patients during hypothermic cardioplegia arrest and normothermic ischemia. *Ann Thorac Surg* 47:663–668, 1989.)

The apparent discrepancy between experimental studies demonstrating a marked tolerance of immature myocardium to ischemia vs. clinical studies implying inadequate myocardial protection as a major cause of postoperative ventricular dysfunction has been difficult to resolve. One explanation may be that, clinically, the myocardium of infants who require surgery within the first few weeks of life is compromised secondary to cyanosis, volume, or pressure overload with associated ventricular hypertrophy and subendocardial ischemia. An alternative explanation may be that the methods of myocardial protection currently used in neonatal cardiac surgery are suboptimal, not because of an inherent greater susceptibility of the immature heart to ischemia but because there are various factors unique to clinical neonatal management that potentiate the damaging effects of cardiopulmonary bypass and the obligatory ischemic period associated with intracardiac repair.

Notwithstanding the critical importance of an accurate and complete anatomical repair in neonatal cardiac surgery, sufficient experimental and clinical data support our impression that myocardial failure attributable to inadequate myocardial protection is an important cause of morbidity and mortality after surgical repair of the newborn heart. In our experience, most infants with severe postoperative low cardiac output have had no residual anatomical lesions, as demonstrated on echocardiographic and catheterization studies, other than marked depression of systolic and diastolic ventricular function. As a consequence, we have attempted to identify the factors that may be responsible for intraoperative injury in the neonatal myocardium and may adversely influence postoperative myocardial function. The potential for damage in the setting of neonatal cardiac surgery may occur at several stages during the operative period: preischemic, ischemic, and reperfusion.

PREISCHEMIC STAGE

Hypothermia

Hypothermia remains the most potent and important protective measure currently available to protect both immature and mature myocardium from the adverse effects of surgically induced ischemia. The reduction in metabolic rate afforded by hypothermia has been well described and is almost universally applied in neonatal myocardial protection strategies. Although the reduction of metabolic processes is clearly beneficial in improving tolerance to ischemia, the slowing of metabolism might itself be harmful and, despite its protective effect, hypothermia, being an essentially unphysiologic state, may also be associated with adverse consequences.

Several years ago, our laboratory became interested in the potentially deleterious effects of hypothermia when we noted that, during cold perfusion on bypass, the infant heart would occasionally become firm and contracted and would remain in a semi-rigid state even after administration of cardioplegia. Invariably, the occurrence of intraoperative "cooling contracture" was associated with severe postoperative low cardiac output syndrome, resulting in significant morbidity and mortality.[12] The term "rapid cooling contracture" refers to a marked increase in resting tension that occurs in both cardiac and skeletal muscle in response to a sudden decrease in temperature.[13] This physiologic phenomenon is well known to muscle physiologists and involves the activation of myofilaments by the release of calcium from intracellular stores in response to a sudden temperature change.[14] Our clinical observations of apparent cold-induced changes in myocardial wall tension were confirmed in isolated perfused neonatal and adult rabbit hearts where preischemic, profoundly hypothermic perfusion induced a marked increase in diastolic pressure and an associated severe depression of postischemic ventricular function.[15, 16]

Similar experimental results documenting the potentially damaging effects of extremely rapid perfusion cooling have been documented by other investigators in myocardial, renal, hepatic, and lung tissue.[17–20] In contrast to our experimental and clinical findings, a number of centers have failed to recognize the cold contracture phenomenon clinically during routine perfusion cooling on bypass. Experimental work from Mayer's laboratory suggests that a reduction in serum levels of ionized calcium during preischemic cooling prevents cooling contracture and may explain why cold-induced myocardial injury is not uniformly observed clinically by other centers whose routine practice includes perfusion cooling on bypass before cardioplegic arrest. We have more recently found that the degree of diastolic tone or resting tension during perfusion cooling in the nonarrested state is related to the absolute level of temperature reduction as well as to the perfusion pressure during cooling, which may further explain why the potentially detrimental effects of hypothermic perfusion occur inconsistently (Fig 2). In isolated perfused neonatal rabbit hearts, we

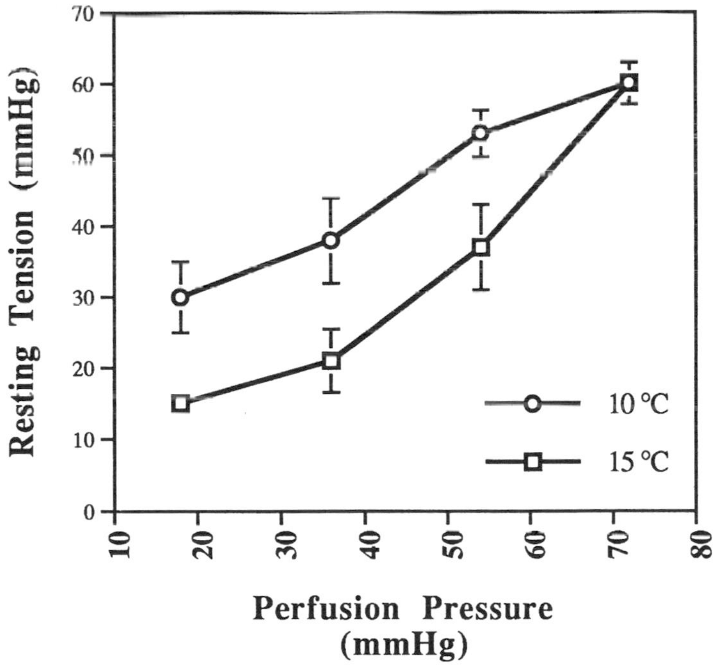

FIGURE 2.

Resting myocardial tension in isolated neonatal rabbit hearts during hypothermic perfusion at varying temperature and coronary perfusion pressure.

found a minimal increase in resting tension when perfusion pressures of less than 40 mm Hg were combined with a perfusate temperature of 15°C. However, an increase in perfusion pressure or reduction in perfusate temperature to 10°C was associated with a significant increase in myocardial resting tension (unpublished data). The mechanisms involved in the interaction between temperature and perfusion pressure in cooling-induced changes in diastolic tone are unknown, but Kitakaze and Marban have demonstrated that both intracellular calcium and contractile force may be modulated by coronary perfusion pressure.[21]

Cooling contracture is therefore not an inevitable consequence of cold perfusion, and hypothermia per se is neither universally beneficial nor harmful; rather, like most therapeutic interventions, it possesses a dose-response curve. Its effect depends on the details of how it is used and under what conditions.

ISCHEMIC STAGE

Calcium Content

Numerous investigators have attempted to determine the optimal calcium concentration in various neonatal cardioplegic solutions. On the basis that calcium overload during ischemia is a major mechanism of myocardial injury, one could argue for the use of either zero or ultralow levels of calcium in cardioplegic formulations; however, continued concern regarding the theoretical potential for calcium paradox has prompted most to avoid acalcemic solutions. Although the neonatal heart is generally believed to be more resistant to the calcium paradox and the concomitant use of hypothermia should even further prevent this form of injury, there are other interacting factors, such as pH, sodium concentration, and duration of ischemia, that potentiate this phenomenon by mechanisms that are not completely understood.[22–24]

Most calcium dose-response studies in which neonatal heart models were used have found that a reduction in the ionized levels of this cation in the cardioplegic solution results in better myocardial recovery.[25–27] Baker has provided detailed studies of this issue in a neonatal rabbit model, thereby suggesting that the calcium content in St. Thomas' II cardioplegic solution may be partially responsible for its purported damaging effect in immature myocardium of this species.[28, 29] In this regard, Hearse has previously shown in adult hearts that the reduction in calcium content in St. Thomas' II solution (1.2 vs. 2.4 mmol) was likely the most important factor for its improved performance compared with St. Thomas' I solution. Torchiana has postulated that hearts remain mechanically active during hyperkalemic arrest and undergo energetically wasteful contraction when perfused with calcium-containing hyperkalemic solutions.[30]

These experimental results support the use of calcium concentrations that are below normal in neonatal cardioplegic solutions. In contrast, several groups have reported that normocalcemic cardioplegia provides better neonatal myocardial protection, but these studies were either performed at normothermia or used excess citrate to reduce ionized calcium, which may have influenced the experimental results.[31–33]

Magnesium

Despite the potential for excessive calcium influx secondary to hyperkalemia-induced membrane depolarization, potassium remains the most widely used arresting agent in neonatal cardiac surgery. Magnesium helps maintain a negative resting membrane potential and competitively inhibits sarcolemmal calcium influx.[34] Accordingly, numerous studies in which adult heart models were used have demonstrated that the addition of magnesium to calcium-containing hyperkalemic cardioplegic solutions improves myocardial preservation.[35–39] Relatively few studies, however, have addressed the potential role of varying levels of magnesium in neonatal cardioplegic solutions. Konishi and Apstein compared three crystalloid cardioplegic solutions with topical hypothermia in a blood perfused neonatal rabbit model and found superior functional recovery with solutions containing magnesium, even though the solution without magnesium was acalcemic.[40] As blood cardioplegic solutions necessarily contain calcium, the addition of magnesium to blood cardioplegia was assessed in a neonatal rabbit model, and a similar beneficial effect was demonstrated.[41]

The magnesium dose-response studies by Hearse and colleagues would suggest that the optimal magnesium concentration for cardioplegic infusates is 16 mmol/L. This "optimal concentration," however, is clearly influenced by temperature and the other components of the cardioplegic formulation, especially calcium. Takemoto et al. studied the calcium–magnesium relationship in cardioplegic solutions and convincingly demonstrated that the cardioprotective effect was dependent on the relative concentrations of both these cations.[42] Further, the interdepedence between magnesium and calcium varied according to the myocardial temperature during ischemia. These complex interactions make it difficult to determine confidently whether magnesium should be a universal addition to all neonatal cardioplegic formulations and at what concentration. What further complicates this issue is the possibility of increased levels of citrate in the cardiopulmonary bypass prime and blood cardioplegia in neonatal cardiac surgery. The standard cardiopulmonary bypass prime used in neonates usually entails addition of stored blood to a crystalloid prime to prevent excessive hemodilution; thus, an obligatory citrate load is imposed on the infant unless fresh, heparinized (i.e., noncitrated) blood is used. The large volume of citrated blood in the bypass circuit in relation to the neonate's circulating blood volume results in serum levels of citrate that far exceed those seen in other clinical settings, especially if fresh frozen plasma is included in the prime composition. We have previously assayed serum levels of citrate on bypass and have found levels reaching 2.0–2.5 mmol/L (or 20–50 times normal) at initiation of bypass. As the use of blood cardioplegia in neonates usually involves the addition of potassium to an aliquot of the bypass prime, the cardioplegic solution itself contains increased levels of citrate by virtue of the citrate present in the prime. Increased serum levels of citrate result in substantial alterations in ionized calcium and magnesium concentrations as a result of its chelating properties. The effect on ionized magnesium is probably even greater, because citrate binds slightly stronger to magnesium than it does the calcium ion.[43] Therefore, elevated levels of citrate in neonatal blood cardioplegic formulations may be potentially detrimental, because the balance between ionized magnesium and calcium is altered.

Single-Dose vs. Multidose Cardioplegic Administration

In the adult heart, the degree of myocardial protection afforded by multidose cardioplegia appears superior to that of single dose cardioplegia or hypothermia alone based on considerable experimental data and clinical experience.[44–46] Accordingly, cardiac surgeons have conventionally administered cardioplegia repeatedly during the course of the ischemic period according to criteria of ischemic duration, myocardial temperature, or the appearance of electrical and mechanical activity. The practice of multidose cardioplegic administration is frequently adopted for use in the neonatal heart, despite experimental and clinical evidence from a number of independent investigators, that, under some conditions, this technique is not as effective and may even be damaging to immature myocardium. Magovern and co-workers initially demonstrated that multidose crystalloid cardioplegia does not provide adequate preservation of hemodynamic function in the immature, as compared with the adult, heart and subsequently showed that both topical hypothermia and single dose cardioplegia were more effective on the basis of postischemic ventricular function indices. These results were confirmed in similar experimental studies by both Sawa and Kohman. DeLeon compared the results of single vs. multidose blood cardioplegia in a series of patients who underwent the arterial switch procedure and found no advantage with multiple administration. Although this clinical study was not randomized, there may have even been a deleterious effect indicated by a higher mortality in the group receiving multidose cardioplegia. The mechanism behind this paradoxical effect of multidose cardioplegia in the neonatal heart is currently unknown. The detailed studies of this phenomenon from Hearse's laboratory suggest that the detrimental effects of multidose hypothermic cardioplegia in the neonatal heart become more evident at infusion temperatures below 20°C and with increasing frequency of administration.[47–49]

POSTISCHEMIC STAGE

Despite increasing evidence that mechanisms of injury occurring during early reperfusion can significantly alter postischemic myocardial function, most congenital cardiac surgeons currently reestablish blood flow to the heart without further manipulating the conditions of reperfusion. Interventions aimed at the reduction of reperfusion–mediated injury include substrate enhancement and ionic modification, free radical scavenging, and leukocyte depletion.[50, 51] Further evidence of their efficacy by independent investigations appears to be necessary, however, before such interventions are adopted into clinical practice. Two relatively simple interventions, however, that are potentially effective and not likely associated with any known adverse effects include the reduction in perfusion pressure and temperature during the initial phase of reperfusion. Studies by Fujiwara and associates in a neonatal lamb heart model have shown that maintaining a low coronary perfusion pressure (i.e., 20 mm Hg) during the initial period of reperfusion was associated with improvement in myocardial and endothelial function.[52] Okada reported in 1988 that transient hypothermia during reoxygenation of the anoxic heart improved contractile recovery and suggested that similar beneficial effects might be attainable with transient hypothermia during postischemic reperfusion.[53] Although Kempsford et al. reported no beneficial effects of transient hypothermic reperfusion on postischemic functional recovery in the isolated rat heart using a range of temperatures, creatine kinase leakage was significantly lower in hearts reperfused at 20°C.[54] Of interest, they demonstrated a marked impairment of myocardial function when hearts were perfused at temperatures below 15°C, as our previous studies on rapid cooling contracture in the rabbit heart have suggested. There was a trend toward increased recovery in hearts reperfused at 20°C although the difference was not statistically significant because of the small group sizes. Although the demonstrated beneficial effects of transient hypothermic and low pressure reperfusion are not striking and remain inconclusive, the simplicity and apparent safety of these interventions makes them appealing to apply in the clinical setting.

NEONATAL MYOCARDIAL PROTECTION: THE HOSPITAL FOR SICK CHILDREN, TORONTO

The myocardial protection techniques currently used at The Hospital for Sick Children in Toronto are based on an integration of experimental data from numerous research laboratories combined with our own clinical observations and experience.

Preischemic Phase

Most neonatal repairs are performed with the use of moderately hypothermic (25°C to 28°C) continuous cardiopulmonary bypass with intermittent periods of low flow ($\approx$ 50 mL/kg/min). Because of continued concern regarding potential neurologic injury, the use of hypothermic circulatory arrest is limited to repair of cardiac lesions requiring aortic arch and anomalous pulmonary venous reconstruction, although short periods of circulatory arrest are also used for portions of the intracardiac repair in infants who weigh less than 5 kg. During the preischemic cooling phase, perfusate temperature is continuously monitored and maintained above 14°C. In contrast to our earlier experience, this method has been uniformly successful in preventing cooling induced myocardial contracture when combined with flow rates of 100 mL/kg/min and corresponding perfusion pressures below 30 mm Hg in the infant. Ionized levels of calcium in the perfusate are only partially corrected at initiation of bypass and are usually in the range of 0.5–0.6 mmol. Previously, the addition of fresh frozen plasma, which contains inordinately high concentrations of citrate, had resulted in ultralow ionized calcium levels of less than 0.05 mmol, which in itself may have been damaging especially during normothermic perfusion. In addition, gas flows are adjusted to maintain pCO_2 levels at 40–45 mm Hg during the cooling phase.

Ischemic Phase

The cardioplegic solution currently used is a 2:1 blood:crystalloid formulation with a hematocrit value of approximately 5%. The base crystalloid solution is a commercially available balanced salt solution (Plasmalyte 148) to which potassium and magnesium are added to obtain a concentration of 16 mmol for both cations in the final mixture. Glucose and bicarbonate are also added, although more recently we have omitted bicarbonate based on studies suggesting that alkalotic cardioplegic solutions may not be as effective in the neonatal heart.[55] The crystalloid component does not contain calcium but, when mixed with the blood perfusate, the ionized calcium concentration in the final cardioplegic solution is approximately 0.6 mmol.

The cardioplegic solution is administered in an anterograde fashion at a dose of 30 mL/kg of body weight. The initial infusion temperature is at or above room temperature but is cooled to 10°C through the cardioplegic heat exchanger as soon as the heart arrests in a flaccid state. Myocardial temperature is continually monitored with a probe, and cardioplegia reinfused if the temperature exceeds 20°C. A specially designed miniature cooling jacket is routinely used and usually maintains myocardial temperature between 12°C to 15°C.

Continuous warm blood cardioplegia is rarely used and is limited to infants who have anomalous origin of the left coronary from the pulmonary artery and are seen with severe left ventricular dysfunction secondary to ongoing ischemia and/or infarction. Continuous retrograde coronary perfusion is maintained at approximately 3–5 mL/kg/min by using a balloon tipped catheter within the coronary sinus along with bicaval venous cannulation to allow for a small right atriotomy incision. The blood cardioplegic temperature is maintained at 28°C to 30°C, and the retrograde flow rate is adjusted depending on the visualization needed to complete reimplantation of the anomalous coronary artery.

Postischemic Phase

Immediately before removal of the aortic cross-clamp, bypass flow rate is reduced to 50% and temperature maintained at 20°C to 25°C for several minutes during the initial reperfusion phase. These simple postischemic interventions do not require complex modifications of the bypass circuit and are potentially beneficial in reducing reperfusion induced injury based on the experimental work noted previously. In addition, ionized levels of calcium are not normalized until myocardial activity has returned and intracardiac monitoring lines have been positioned in preparation for separation from bypass.

RESULTS

Review of our clinical results during the past several years has demonstrated a significant improvement in postoperative morbid-

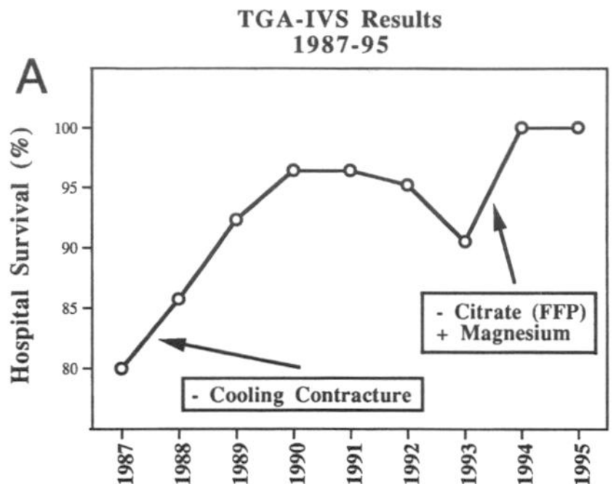

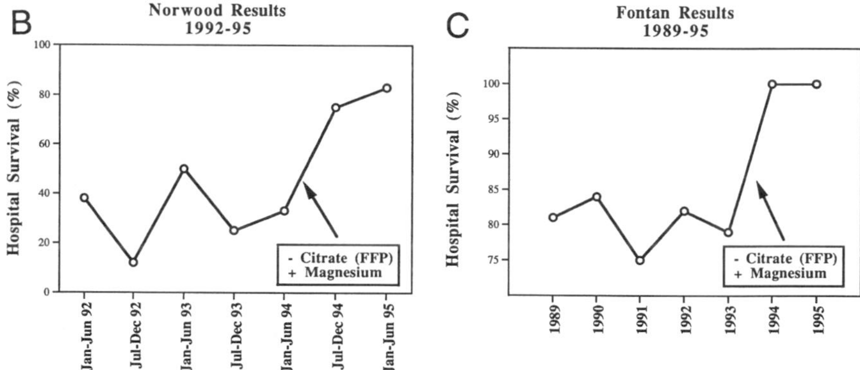

FIGURE 3.
Trends in hospital survival (%) for the arterial switch procedure for transposition with intact ventricular septum **(A)**, the Norwood procedure **(B)**, and the Fontan procedure **(C)** in relation to modifications in myocardial protection techniques.

ity and mortality that can be, at least partially, attributed to modifications of our myocardial protection techniques. Review of the hospital survival for the arterial switch procedure for transposition of the great arteries with intact ventricular septum reveals that, before our recognition of the potentially adverse consequences of rapid cooling contracture, we experienced hospital mortality rates of 20% (Fig 3A). By eliminating this negative influence, hospital survival rate increased to 90% to 95%. A subsequent improvement in hospital survival was experienced in mid-1994 after further modifications, including the removal of fresh frozen plasma from the cardiopulmonary bypass prime to reduce circulating (and cardioplegic) citrate levels and the addition of magnesium to the blood cardioplegic formulation.

The change in clinical results was even more evident in hospital survival rates for the Norwood procedure during the same period (Fig 3B). Before mid-1994, we had experienced excessively high mortality rates with this operation, which we attributed to early postoperative ventricular dysfunction despite the acknowledgment of the technically demanding aspects of the Norwood procedure. Similarly, the improvement in our neonatal surgical clinical results was translated to other age groups on the basis of our experience with the Fontan operation (Fig 3C). Postoperative mortality rates had remained relatively constant at 15% to 20% until 1994, when a significant change in both morbidity and mortality occurred. The superior results may have also been affected by our change to the almost exclusive use of either the "lateral tunnel" and "extracardiac" method of performing the Fontan procedure. In addition, pre-Fontan staging with a bidirectional cavopulmonary anastomosis probably had a positive effect.

CONCLUSIONS

In summary, our experimental and clinical observations have taught us that effective neonatal myocardial protection involves more than simply arresting the heart with a high potassium solution and cooling it as much as possible. Methods of myocardial protection successfully used in some centers may yield drastically different results when applied by others, because of seemingly small dissimilarities in intraoperative technique and protocol. Experimental studies have repeatedly demonstrated that relatively minor changes in cardioplegic formulation and application can have major effects on the effectiveness of myocardial preservation, which reveals the major gaps in our understanding of the mechanisms of injury and protection. The application of information derived from laboratory-based research combined with clinical observation has allowed us to mitigate what had been a major source of morbidity and mortality and has highlighted the importance of critically assessing one's results and carefully probing for potentially adverse factors. It is therefore realistic to conclude that preservation of postoperative myocardial function is of paramount importance in determining neonatal surgical results, second only to the technical aspects of a precise and complete surgical repair.

REFERENCES

1. Groom RC, Hill AG, Akl BF, et al: Pediatric perfusion survey. *Proc Am Acad Cardiovasc Perfusion* 11:78–84, 1990.
2. Bull C, Stark J: Cardioplegic protection of the child's heart. *J Thorac Cardiovasc Surg* 88:287–293, 1984.
3. Hammon J, Graham T, Boucek R, et al: Myocardial adenosine triphos-

phate content as a measure of metabolic and functional myocardial protection in children undergoing cardiac operation. *Ann Thorac Surg* 44:467–470, 1987.

4. Lofland G, Abd-Elfattah A, Wyse R, et al: Myocardial adenine nucleotide metabolism in pediatric patients during hypothermic cardioplegia arrest and normothermic ischemia. *Ann Thorac Surg* 47:633–638, 1989.
5. Grice W, Konishi T, Apstein C: Resistance of neonatal myocardium to injury during normothermic and hypothermic ischemic arrest and reperfusion. *Circulation* 76(suppl V):150–155, 1987.
6. Jarmakani J, Nakazawa M, Nagatomo T, et al: Effect of hypoxia on mechanical function in the neonatal mammalian heart. *Am J Physiol* 235:469H–474H, 1978.
7. Murphy C, Salter D, Morris J, et al: Age-related differences in adenine nucleotide metabolism during in vivo global ischemia. *Surg Forum* 37:288–290, 1986.
8. Yano Y, Braimbridge MV, Hearse DJ: Protection of the pediatric myocardium. *J Thorac Cardiovasc Surg* 94:887–896, 1986.
9. Wittnich C, Peniston C, Ianuzzo D, et al: Relative vulnerability of neonatal and adult hearts to ischemic injury. *Circulation* 76(suppl V):156–160, 1987.
10. Parrish M, Payne A, Fixler D: Global myocardial ischemia in the newborn, juvenile, and adult isolated isovolumic rabbit heart. *Circ Res* 61:609–615, 1987.
11. Pridjian AK, Levitsky S, Krukenkamp I, et al: Developmental changes in reperfusion injury: Comparison of intracelllular ion accumulation in ischemic and cardioplegic arrest. *J Thorac Cardiovasc Surg* 96:577–581, 1988.
12. Williams WG, Rebeyka IM, Tibshirani RJ, et al: Warm induction blood cardioplegia in the infant. *J Thorac Cardiovasc Surg* 100(6):896–901, 1990.
13. Sakai T, Kurihara S: The rapid cooling contracture of toad cardiac muscles. *Jpn J Physiol* 24:649–666, 1974.
14. Konishi M, Kurihara S, Sakai T: Change in intracellular calcium ion concentration induced by caffeine and rapid cooling in frog skeletal muscle fibres. *J Physiol* 365:131–146, 1985.
15. Rebeyka IM, Hanan SA, Borges MR, et al: Rapid cooling contracture of the myocardium: The adverse effect of pre-arrest cardiac hypothermia. *J Thorac Cardiovasc Surg* 100:240–249, 1990.
16. Rebeyka IM, Diaz RJ, Augustine JM, et al: Effect of rapid cooling contracture on ischemic tolerance in immature myocardium. *Circulation* 84(suppl III):III-389–III-393, 1991.
17. Jynge P: Protection of the ischemic myocardium: Cold chemical cardioplegia, coronary infustates and the importance of cellular calcium control. *Thorac Cardiovasc Surgeon* 28:310–321, 1980.
18. Jacobsen IB, Kemp E, Buhl MR: An adverse effect of rapid cooling in kidney transplantation. *Transplantation* 27:135–136, 1979.

19. Otto G, Wolff H, Uerlings I, et al: Preservation damage in liver transplantation. *Transplantation* 42(2):122–124, 1986.
20. Wang L-S, Nakamoto K, Hsieh C-M, et al: Influence of temperature of flushing solution on lung preservation. *Ann Thorac Surg* 55:711–715, 1993.
21. Kitakaze M, Marban E: Cellular mechanism of the modulation of contractile function by coronary perfusion pressure in ferret hearts. *J Physiol* 414:455–472, 1989.
22. Uemura S, Young H, Matsuoka S, et al: Calcium paradox in the neonatal heart. *Can J Cardiol* 1:114–120, 1985.
23. Chapman RA, Suleiman MS, Rodrigo GC, et al: The calcium paradox: A role for [Na]i, a cellular or tissue basis, a property unique to the Langendorff perfused heart? A bundle of contradictions! *J Mol Cell Cardiol* 23:773–777, 1991.
24. Holland CEJ, Olson RE: Prevention by hypothermia of paradoxical calcium necrosis in cardiac muscle. *J Mol Cell Cardiol* 7:917–928, 1975.
25. Caspi J, Herman SL, Coles JG, et al: Effects of low perfusate Ca++ concentration on newborn myocardial function after ischemia. *Circulation* 82(suppl IV):IV-371–IV-379, 1990.
26. Robinson LA: Calcium in neonatal cardioplegia. *Ann Thorac Surg* 51:1043–1044, 1991.
27. Riva E, Hearse DJ: Calcium and cardioplegia in neonates: Dose-response and time-response studies in rats. *Am J Physiol* 261:1609H–1616H, 1991.
28. Baker EJI, Olinger GN, Baker JE: Calcium content of St. Thomas' II cardioplegic solution damages ischemic immature myocardium. *Ann Thorac Surg* 52:993–999, 1991.
29. Baker EJ, Baker JE: Calcium and cardioplegic protection of the ischemic immature heart: Impact of hypoxemia from birth. *Ann Thorac Surg* 58:1123–1130, 1994.
30. Torchiana DF, Love TR, Hendren WG, et al: Calcium-induced ventricular contraction during cardioplegic arrest. *J Thorac Cardiovasc Surg* 94:606–613, 1987.
31. Zweng TN, Iannettoni MD, Bove EL, et al: The concentration of calcium in neonatal cardioplegia. *Ann Thorac Surg* 50:262–267, 1990.
32. Pearl JM, Laks H, Drinkwater DC, et al: Normocalcemic blood or crystalloid cardioplegia provides superior neonatal myocardial protection over low calcium cardioplegia. *AATS Meeting* 1993, pp 54–55.
33. Corno A, Bethencourt D, Laks H, et al: Myocardial protection in the neonatal heart. *J Thorac Cardiovasc Surg* 92(2):163–172, 1987.
34. Kraft LF, Katholi RE, Woods WT, et al: Attenuation by magnesium of the electrophysiologic effects of hyperkalemia on human and canine heart cells. *Am J Cardiol* 45:1189–1195, 1980.
35. Hearse D, Stewart D, Braimbridge M: Myocardial protection during ischemic cardiac arrest: The importance of magnesium in cardioplegic infusates. *J Thorac Cardiovasc Surg* 75:877–885, 1978.
36. Geffin GA, Love TR, Hendren WG, et al: The effects of calcium and

magnesium in hyperkalemic solutions on myocardial preservation. *J Thorac Cardiovasc Surg* 98:239–250, 1989.
37. Wakabayashi A, Nishi T, Guilmette J: Experimental evaluation of magnesium cardioplegia. *J Thorac Cardiovasc Surg* 84:685–688, 1982.
38. Reynolds TR, Geffin GA, Titus JS, et al: Myocardial preservation related to magnesium content of hyperkalemic cardioplegic solution at 8°C. *Ann Thorac Surg* 47:907–913, 1989.
39. Brown P, Holland F, Parenteau G, et al: Magnesium ion is essential in crystalloid cardioplegia. *J Mol Cell Cardiol* 22(suppl V):S.3, 1990.
40. Konishi T, Apstein CS: Comparison of three cardioplegic solutions during hypothermic ischemic arrest in neonatal blood perfused rabbit hearts. *J Thorac Cardiovasc Surg* 98:1132–1137, 1989.
41. Rebeyka IM, Diaz RM, Waddell JF, et al: Magnesium-based blood cardioplegia in a neonatal heart model. *Circulation* 86(suppl I):I-630, 1992.
42. Takemoto N, Kuroda H, Hamasaki T, et al: Effect of magnesium and calcium on myocardial protection by cardioplegic solutions. *Ann Thorac Surg* 57:177–182, 1994.
43. Dzik W, Kikrley S: Citrate toxicity during massive blood transfusion. *Transfus Med Rev* 2:76–94, 1988.
44. Engelman RM, Auvil J, O'Donoghue MJ, et al: The significance of multidose cardioplegia and hypothermia in myocardial preservation during ischemic arrest. *J Thorac Cardiovasc Surg* 75:555–563, 1978.
45. Lucas SK, Elmer EB, Flaherty JT, et al: Effect of multiple-dose potassium cardioplegia on myocardial ischemia, return of ventricular function, and ultrastructural preservation. *J Thorac Cardiovasc Surg* 80:102–110, 1980.
46. Daily PO, Jones B, Folkerth TL, et al: Comparison of myocardial temperatures with multidose cardioplegia versus single dose cardioplegia and myocardial surface cooling during coronary artery bypass grafting. *J Thorac Cardiovasc Surg* 97:715–724, 1989.
47. Kempsford RD, Hearse DJ: Protection of the immature heart. *J Thorac Cardiovasc Surg* 99:269–279, 1990.
48. Murashita T, Avkiran M, Hearse DJ: Detrimental effects of multidose hypothermic cardioplegia in the neonatal heart: The role of frequency of cardioplegia infusions. *Eur J Cardiothorac Surg* 5:183–190, 1991.
49. Murashita T, Hearse DJ: Temperature-response studies of the detrimental effects of multidose versus single-dose cardioplegic solution in the rabbit heart. *J Thorac Cardiovasc Surg* 102:673–683, 1991.
50. Follette DM, Fey K, Buckberg GD, et al: Reducing postischemic damage by temporary modification of reperfusate calcium, potassium, pH, and osmolarity. *J Thorac Cardiovasc Surg* 82:221–238, 1981.
51. Kawata H, Sawatari K, Mayer JEJ: Evidence for the role of neutrophils in reperfusion injury after cold cardioplegic ischemia in neonatal lambs. *J Thorac Cardiovasc Surg* 103:908–918, 1992.
52. Fujiwara T, Kurtts T, Silvera M, et al: Physical and pharmacological

manipulations of reperfusion conditions in neonatal myocardial preservation. *Circulation* 78:II-444, 1988.

53. Okada T: Facilitating effect of cold shock on recovery from anoxia-induced contractile depression in isolated rat heart and heart muscle. *Circ Res* 62:338–346, 1988.
54. Kempsford RD, Murashita T, Hearse DJ: Transient hypothermic reperfusion and postischemic recovery in isolated rat heart. *Am J Physiol* 259:879H–888H, 1990.
55. Iannettoni MD, Bove EL, Fox MH, et al: The effect of intramyocardial pH on functional recovery in neonatal hearts receiving St. Thomas' Hospital cardioplegic solution during global ischemia. *J Thorac Cardiovasc Surg* 104:333–343, 1992.

Coagulation in Cardiac Surgery

D. Royston, F.R.C.A.
Consultant in Cardiothoracic Anaesthesia, Harefield Hospital, Middlesex, England

It is now more than ten years since I obtained Ethical Committee approval to study the effects of very high doses of aprotinin given to patients for a short period while they were having open heart surgery. During the subsequent years, the efficacy of aprotinin and other serine protease inhibitors has been shown in a large number of studies and in different forms of surgery.[1–3]

Since its introduction to the market, there has been a continuous undercurrent of the "controlled anecdote," suggesting dangers or problems with aprotinin therapy. This undercurrent is similar to that seen with a number of other innovations and therapeutic strategies developed outside North America. Examples include reports of increased mortality with the use of a relaxant-based anesthetic technique[4] and reports indicating that the preoperative administration of β-adrenoreceptor antagonists is directly associated with mortality after cardiac surgery.[5] The best example is a study of halothane hepatotoxicity that showed a significant problem by retrospectively including data from centers that had reported a potential problem after use of halothane anesthesia.[6] Many of the claimed deleterious effects of aprotinin therapy have failed to materialize during controlled clinical trials. This does not mean that there are no bad effects of aprotinin therapy but, more likely, that these effects are less biologically relevant to most clinicians. The greatest problem associated with overcoming these accusations is that the precise mechanism of action of the agent is unknown.

In this review, I address three major topics related to aprotinin and other serine protease inhibitors. First, I will demonstrate that the serine protease inhibitors are not simply an expensive form of the lysine analogues epsilon-amino caproic acid and tranexamic acid. Aprotinin and the serine protease inhibitors have an entirely separate spectrum of efficacy and toxicity/adverse effects. The most obvious of these effects is the potential for an adverse reaction to occur after a second exposure to aprotinin. The second topic ad-

© 1996, Mosby–Year Book, Inc.

dressed will be how aprotinin may work. In this section, I also discuss the intriguing possibility that increasing anticoagulation will prevent the hemostatic defect associated with cardiac surgery and thus reduce postoperative bleeding. Finally, I will examine a number of the adverse effects that have been laid at the feet of high-dose aprotinin therapy.

IS APROTININ JUST AN EXPENSIVE FORM OF AMICAR?

HOW DO WE MEASURE THE INHIBITION OF FIBRINOLYSIS?

The first question to address is the definition of an antifibrinolytic agent and the end point that you choose to suggest that fibrinolysis has been inhibited. At first, this may seem remarkably simple to answer, but further consideration will produce some confusion.

In most test systems, the plasma concentration of split products of fibrin is measured. If there is a reduction in the concentration of these split products, it is assumed that an antifibrinolytic agent has been administered. As we have increased our understanding of the molecular structure of fibrinogen and its degradation, the tests of this fibrinolytic activity have become more specific, complex, and expensive.

Earlier methods of measurement determined whether split products of fibrin were present in a system by using relatively crude but effective turbidity methods. It is now possible to measure specific fragments released during the breakdown of fibrin and, particularly, the concentration of substances such as the D-dimer fragment. As discussed later in this article, the finding of lower plasma concentrations of D-dimer does not solely imply a specific antifibrinolytic activity of an agent. For there to be fibrinolysis, fibrin must obviously be generated in a site, such as the blood stream, that can be lysed. It is intuitively obvious that if there is no generation of fibrin then there will be no split products to measure.

DO ALL ANTIFIBRINOLYTICS INHIBIT "NATURAL" FIBRINOLYSIS EQUALLY?

This question is of crucial importance when considering whether to use an agent that is thought to act solely as an inhibitor of natural lysis. For the cardiac surgeon and other surgeons, it is imperative that if fibrin is formed in either an abnormal amount or in an abnormal position, then this fibrin will be dissolved and will not lead to occlusion of the microvasculature. One of the most intriguing aspects of the use of agents purported to inhibit fibrinolysis is their lack of effect on normal "baseline" fibrinolysis. All currently used methods of measuring split products of fibrin, such as D-dimer, have a normal range. Indeed, all publications on this subject show baseline control data with a mean and variance for these variables for the patient population being studied. It is of interest that these values have never been reported to decrease after administration of an inhibitor of fibrinolysis alone. Does this imply that there is a part of the normal fibrinolytic process that we cannot inhibit with available pharmaceutical interventions? Or, does it mean that these particular assays are not as specific as we would hope?

Notwithstanding these comments, a number of interesting data come from various in vivo and in vitro studies of the effects of certain antifibrinolytic drugs to inhibit the dissolution of fibrin induced after administration of naturally occurring agents, such as tissue plasminogen activator (t-PA) or single-chain urokinase-type plasminogen activator (scuPA).

The first set of data comparing lysine analogues with aprotinin is from studies in which investigators were looking for methods to inhibit fibrinolytic drugs administered for their therapeutic action.[7] In these studies, the lytic agent was added to pre-formed blood clot, and the rate of lysis was measured. These methods were then repeated with the addition of various proposed inhibitors of the process. The results of the studies suggested that administration of the lysine analogues would produce a 100% inhibition of lysis produced by t-PA. In contrast, aprotinin produced only approximately 50% inhibition of this lytic activity. The results of these laboratory studies would suggest that if fibrin were formed, then the process of lysis would be totally inhibited by the lysine analogues but would still progress, albeit more slowly, in the presence of aprotinin therapy.

This line of thought is supported by placebo-controlled studies of the effects of aprotinin therapy in patients undergoing cardiopulmonary bypass.[8] As part of the studies, plasma samples from these patients were collected to perform a measurement termed the euglobin clot lysis test. For this test, the patient's plasma was treated to remove naturally occurring inhibitors of fibrinolysis and was placed onto pre-prepared fibrin plates. After a set period, the area of dissolution or lysis of fibrin on the plate was measured, giving an index of the potential fibrinolytic activity of the plasma. The data from these studies are shown in Figure 1. During cardiopulmonary bypass, there is a decrease in the ability of the plasma to lyse fibrin plates in patients who have received aprotinin therapy. It is also obvious, however, that after administration of protamine,

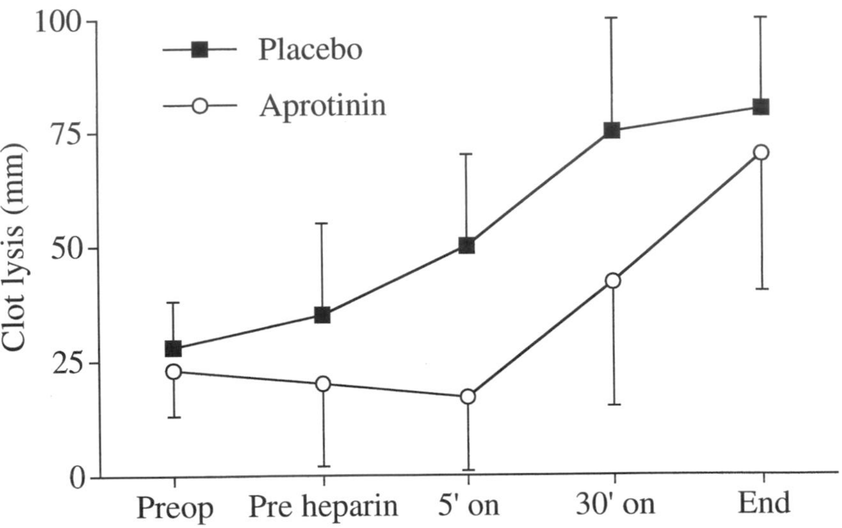

FIGURE 1.
The data (mean ± SD) show the area of lysis of fibrin plates produced by the euglobin fraction of plasma from patients having primary coronary artery bypass graft. During bypass, there is a significant difference in fibrinolytic activity between aprotinin and placebo groups. At the end of bypass, fibrinolytic activity was the same for both groups. (Adapted from Dietrich W, Spannagl M, Jochum M, et al: Influence of high-dose aprotinin treatment on blood loss and coagulation patterns in patients undergoing myocardial revascularization. *Anesthesiology* 73:1119–1126, 1990.)

the natural fibrinolytic activity in the plasma has not been reduced by the aprotinin therapy and is the same as that in the control group. These data support in vitro data and suggest that the natural process of fibrinolysis is not prevented by the use of high-dose aprotinin therapy.

The question arising from the data concerns the mechanism of reduced lytic activity during the bypass. One option is that this reduced clot lysis time during surgery reflects the known inhibitory activity of aprotinin toward plasmin.[9, 10] A second suggestion would be that the natural initiators of the fibrinolytic system, such as t-PA and scUPA, were not released in the presence of aprotinin. This may be because there was (1) less contact activation with reduced generation of kallikrein, which is necessary for the release of scUPA[11, 12]; or (2) less release of t-PA. The release of t-PA from the endothelium is initiated by thrombin, bradykinin, and various cytokines.[13, 14] Administration of aprotinin is associated with reduced generation of cytokines such as interleukin-6 during cardiac surgery.[15, 16] Reduced contact activation should lead to reduced release of bradykinin,[17] and generation of thrombin is less with the use of aprotinin therapy.[18–20] This topic is discussed in greater detail later in this article.

DO ALL ANTIFIBRINOLYTIC DRUGS HAVE THE SAME SPECTRUM OF ACTIVITY TO INHIBIT BLEEDING?

Thus far, reports in the literature suggest that serine protease inhibitors such as aprotinin have a far greater range of activity in terms of efficacy and variety of operative procedures than do the lysine analogue antifibrinolytics. In addition to the benefits associated with open heart surgery and, particularly, complex open heart surgery, aprotinin has been shown[22–27] to have benefits during heart and lung transplantation in patients with endocarditis[2, 21] and in patients who require prolonged extracorporeal support, such as in extracorporeal membrane oxygenation and ventricular assist device support.[28, 29] Nafamostat (FUT-175) has also shown benefits in reducing bleeding in these circumstances.[30] Patients who receive aspirin before surgery have a tendency to have abnormally high blood loss, which can be inhibited with high-dose aprotinin therapy.[31–33] Aprotinin has been shown to be effective in thrombocytopenic states.[34] It has also been shown to reduce bleeding in other situations. Its use has been particularly successful in patients who require emergency surgery after thrombolytic therapy[35–37] and in patients who are taking oral anticoagulants up to the time of surgery.[38] There have been many reports of the efficacy of other serine protease inhibitors to reduce the bleeding associated with prolonged extracorporeal circulation such as hemodialysis.[39, 40] These therapies—especially aprotinin therapy—have also been used to prevent bleeding associated with vascular surgery,[41, 42] liver transplant surgery,[43–47] orthopedic surgery,[48, 49] and neurosurgery[50–52] and, also, in obstetric practice.[53, 54]

The reason for this greater spectrum of activity is probably a result of the difference in the mechanism of action of the agents. Serine protease inhibitors such as aprotinin are precisely what their name implies: inhibitors of certain enzymes. To exert an antifibrinolytic action, aprotinin will inhibit plasmin. There are many other enzymes in biologically controlled processes that are also inhibited by aprotinin.[9] In contrast, the lysine analogue antifibrinolytics act by binding to lysine on plasminogen. Therefore, free plasminogen is not activated by enzymatic degradation by plasminogen activators.[10, 55, 56]

The difference in the effectiveness of these two groups of compounds is probably best described by considering data from animal studies in which ways to inhibit bleeding induced by therapeutic interventions with agents such as t-PA were investigated. In one such study, it was possible to increase the bleeding tendency, as shown by an increase in the bleeding time from a cut wound, with the administration of t-PA. This increased bleeding time is presumed to be a consequence of increased fibrinolysis. In this model, the administration of the lysine analogue tranexamic acid before t-PA showed no effect on bleeding time. In contrast, aprotinin reduced bleeding time to near normal values.[57] These data are expressed in the graph in Figure 2. Presumably, the ability of apro-

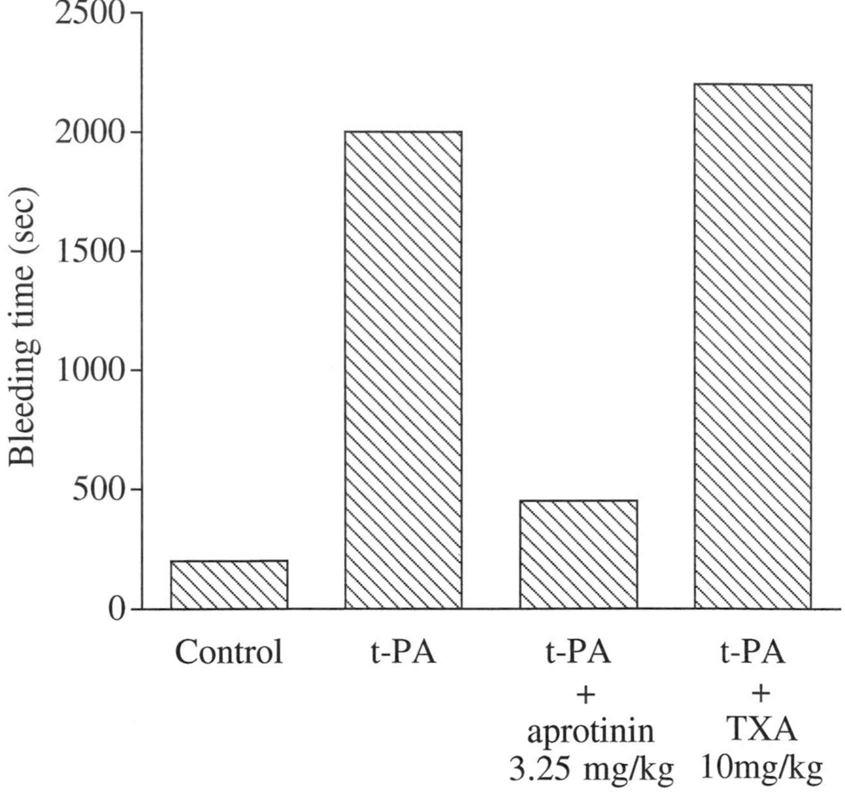

FIGURE 2.

Results for bleeding time in an animal model of fibrinolysis induced by administration of tissue type plasminogen activator (t-PA). The prolonged bleeding time is reversed by co-administration of aprotinin (3.25 mg/kg or 20,0000 kIU/kg) but is not affected by the co-administration of tranexamic acid (10 mg/kg). (Adapted from de Bono D, Pringle S, Underwood I: Differential effects of aprotinin and tranexamic acid on cerebral bleeding and cutaneous bleeding time during rt-PA infusion. *Thromb Res* 61:159–163, 1991.)

tinin to return the hemostatic process to a more normal level is unrelated to its antifibrinolytic action; otherwise, there should have been some evidence for efficacy of tranexamic acid. These data suggest that aprotinin can inhibit bleeding by a mechanism unrelated to its effect on fibrinolysis.

DO APROTININ AND THE LYSINE ANALOGUES HAVE THE SAME SPECTRUM OF SIDE EFFECTS?

The lysine analogues and aprotinin have different chemistry, pharmacokinetic, pharmacodynamic, and safety profiles.[58] In terms of the safety profile, the difference between the two types of agents is best seen by considering the action of these agents on the brain and cerebral circulation. Several early studies conducted in Europe in the late 1960s and early 1970s examined the role of various drug therapies in patients who had a ruptured cerebral artery aneurysm leading to a subarachnoid hemorrhage (SAH).

Administration of either aprotinin or tranexamic acid, or both, was associated with a reduction in the rate of rebleeding seen with this pathology. Later studies suggested, however, that the mortality from SAH in patients given tranexamic acid was not reduced, as these groups of patients had an increase in cerebral ischemia resulting from increased cerebral vasospasm.[59, 60] Indeed, the administration of tranexamic and ϵ-aminocaproic acids over short periods has been noted to be associated with spontaneous arterial thrombosis.[61–63] The lack of any increase in the reporting of such problems in patients undergoing cardiac surgery may be caused by a number of reasons. First, tranexamic acid may have this effect only after prolonged (more than 48 hours) administration. Second, tranexamic acid may not adversely effect blood flow without the presence of a severe perturbation, such as SAH. A further, alternate explanation is that the incidence of cerebral artery vasospasm is considerably reduced by calcium channel antagonists,[64] agents that are commonly used in patients undergoing myocardial revascularization.

In contrast, there is now a considerable body of evidence to show that serpins can greatly modify cerebral blood flow, possibly through an action on kallikrein. These agents relieve the cerebral vessel vasospasm that accompanies SAH.[65–67] This finding has led to the suggestion that aprotinin should be given in combination with epsilon aminocaproic acid to reduce the incidence of cerebral ischemia associated with lysine analogues without increasing the rate of rebleeding.[62, 68]

Recent studies have also shown that cerebral edema is reduced by aprotinin after a prolonged period of ischemia in an animal model of cerebral injury.[69] This is associated with a preservation of the intermediate energy metabolites, such as adenosine 5′-diphosphate and adenosine triphosphate.

In the clinical setting of heart surgery, 670 patients were treated with high-dose aprotinin as part of an open-label study in the United Kingdom. Only 3 patients were noted to have stroke and neurologic deficit.[3, 70] More than 400 of these patients were undergoing reoperation surgery, and nearly 80 had septic endocarditis at the time of their surgery. This incidence of stroke of less than half of 1% is strikingly different from the 3% to 6% incidence reported from other centers[71, 72] where this group of patients was not given aprotinin.

That aprotinin therapy may be associated with a reduced incidence of cerebral complications after open heart surgery has also been shown in patients undergoing primary[73] and reoperation[74] cardiac revascularization. Indeed, in this second report, the incidence of stroke in patients receiving aprotinin therapy was significantly ($P < 0.01$) reduced compared with that in patients in the control group.

There are other obvious differences in the potential anti-inflammatory actions of the two classes of compounds. Aprotinin, like all serine protease inhibitors, has marked anti-inflammatory actions that may be of additional benefit in patients undergoing major surgery—especially open heart surgery.[75, 76]

In summary, the wider spectrum and degree of activity of high-dose aprotinin, coupled with its beneficial effects on hemostasis, imply a completely different mode of action to prevent the need for donor blood than what has been shown with the lysine analogue–type agents. In addition, other studies have suggested that if fibrin formation *does* occur, then aprotinin therapy will not totally prevent the dissolution of such a clot. The results of the one study done in cardiac surgery patients thus far suggest that the process of natural fibrinolysis is not inhibited by aprotinin therapy during the period immediately after bypass.

MECHANISM OF ACTION

There has been much controversy regarding the precise mechanism of action of aprotinin, largely because there is no consensus as to how exactly the hemostatic process works during normal and stressful situations. The three potential mechanisms can be broadly divided into the following:

- Preservation of platelet function. There is much evidence of the ability of serine protease inhibitors to inhibit platelet activation. However, other drugs with less efficacy to inhibit bleeding also show this effect.[58]
- Reduction of fibrinolysis. This aspect is discussed above and in other reviews on this topic.[2, 3]
- Inhibition of generation of thrombin. There is considerable evidence to show that reduced generation of thrombin may be of benefit in patients undergoing open heart surgery.[11, 75]

Can an increase in anticoagulation lead to a decrease in bleeding after cardiac surgery? This obvious paradox is something that many clinicians find difficult to comprehend. Surgeons who have used high-dose aprotinin therapy, however, will comment that the patient looked remarkably dry but that there was also very little evidence of clot formation.

In addition to the many studies of the effects of aprotinin, two other studies have suggested that the hemostatic defect associated with cardiopulmonary bypass is reduced or prevented in patients who have an apparent increase in anticoagulation during bypass. The first study, from 1986, involved the use of prostacyclin.[77] The authors showed an increase in the activated clotting time (ACT) during bypass. This increase presumably was the result of a known effect of prostacyclin on platelet function.[78] It is also well recognized that platelet numbers and function significantly alter the duration of ACT.[79] Notwithstanding this mechanism of action, the ACT measurement principle reflects the final production of fibrin and a coagulum in the analysis tube. Therefore, formation of fibrin as the end point must be regarded as coagulation, and an increase in the ACT must be considered an index of anticoagulation. In this study of the effects of prostacyclin, there was also a statistically significant decrease in the requirements for donor blood. The car diovascular effects of prostacyclin, however, were such that the authors believed the drug was not likely to be of great benefit in clinical practice.

A second, more recent study from Despotis and the group in St. Louis[80] showed that administration of an increased dose of heparin to achieve a target heparin concentration of approximately 6 IU/mL throughout the bypass procedure was associated with decreased consumption of coagulation factors and decreases in the concentration of plasma fibrinopeptide A (FPA) and thrombin-antithrombin III (TAT) complex concentrations. Of most interest

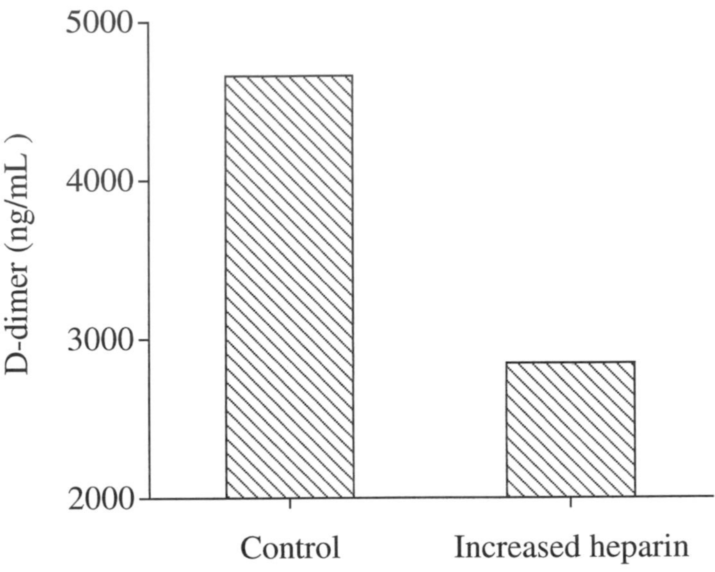

FIGURE 3.

Results for the concentration of the D-dimer product of fibrin breakdown. Mean results are shown from data of Despotis et al.[80] Reduced fibrin formation with higher doses of heparin are reflected in the reduced ($P < 0.05$) concentration of D-dimer.

was a significant reduction in the plasma concentration of D-dimers in patients who had received the higher dose heparin regimen (Fig 3). Unless there is some evidence of which I am not aware, there is, in my opinion, no suggestion that heparin is an antifibrinolytic drug. The concentration of D-dimers must have been reduced because there was less fibrin to dissolve as a result of reduced thrombin generation and activity.

Numerous studies have shown that aprotinin therapy will cause prolongation of the ACT.[3] Whether this is a result of the effects of aprotinin on platelets or on the coagulation cascade is unclear. Studies in human beings have also shown that generation of markers of the coagulation process is decreased in patients who have received aprotinin therapy.[8, 18–20, 81] In particular, investigators have measured concentrations of FPA, prothrombin fragment 1.2, and the TAT complex.

The most intriguing data on the possible mechanism of action of aprotinin, however, come from investigations of the effects of three separate drug therapies (prostacyclin, aprotinin, and increased heparin) on the hemostatic process, as shown by the post-

TABLE 1.
Effect of Different Interventions on Mean Values for Bleeding Time (min) in Early Postoperative Period

	Control/Placebo	Treatment	*P*	Reference
Prostacyclin	8.6	5.5	<0.05	77
Aprotinin	9.8	5.4	<0.05	21
High-dose heparin	8.4	5.9	<0.05	80

operative bleeding time. Many authorities would suggest that the bleeding time is one of the better methods of assessing the overall function of the hemostatic process. Past studies have suggested that the bleeding time is prolonged after a period of open heart surgery.[82] Table 1 shows the bleeding times for untreated patients and those receiving the treatment with one of the three aforementioned modalities to prolong the activated coagulation process. In the three instances where coagulation was improved, as shown by a prolongation in the ACT, there was a significant benefit of normalizing the bleeding time in these patients in the early postoperative period. This observation is intriguing, but I believe it will be remarkably difficult to persuade our clinical colleagues to accept the view that preventing clotting will in some way prevent postoperative bleeding in patients undergoing open heart surgery. It does, however, lead to the possibility that other, more specific antithrombin agents that are being produced may have significant benefit toward improving patient outcome with regard to bleeding after cardiac surgery.

ADVERSE EFFECTS OF APROTININ THERAPY

Thus far, there have been no pharmacologic interventions that have had 100% benefit and no associated risk. Aprotinin is no different in this regard. The various aspects of the adverse events that could be attributed to aprotinin therapy, however, have been like continuously shifting sands over the past few years. The largest problem addressed during that period was how to persuade clinicians that aprotinin is not a procoagulant substance. This subject has been the focus of a number of extensive reviews that have outlined the known pharmacologic reasons why this process should not occur and have explained the current controlled data investigating graft patency in patients who are having both primary and re-operation coronary artery bypass surgery.

GRAFT PATENCY AND THROMBOTIC RISK

Discussion of the effects of drug therapies on graft function should be viewed against the 'normal' or 'expected' rates of graft occlusion in patients having myocardial revascularization. In three recent reports from large studies, the rate of vein graft occlusion, demonstrated by angiographic techniques, was between 5% and 13%.[83–85]

The results for graft occlusion in four placebo-controlled studies[86–89] in which aprotinin therapy was administered to the patients are shown in Table 2. In patients given aprotinin therapy, there was no significant effect of the drug on the incidence of graft occlusions. Current evidence suggests that aprotinin has no clinically significant effect on graft thrombosis.

However, investigators at one center that participated in the multicenter study, reported by Lemmer et al.,[89] did suggest a possible deleterious effect of aprotinin on graft patency.[90] This group specifically addressed the problems of a poor target vessel. Graft occlusions were more likely when there was a poor target vessel. This observation is entirely in keeping with the impression and practice of all clinicians. Large, multicenter studies from Europe[85, 91] showed that graft occlusion was more likely depending on the condition and diameter of the target vessel. It also was of interest that despite graft occlusions being recognized in aprotinin-treated patients, there was no associated evidence of myocardial infarction or additional myocardial ischemia.[90]

Another factor that may have played a part in the reports of a

TABLE 2.
Results From Four Placebo-controlled Studies of the Effects of "High-dose" Aprotinin Therapy on Coronary Artery Bypass Graft Patency

	Control		Aprotinin	
	Occluded	Total	Occluded	Total
Bidstrup et al.[86]	4	138	5	131
Havel et al.[87]	3	40	2	39
Lass et al.[88]	13	102	13	124
Lemmer et al.[89]	8	163	14	176
Total	**28**	**443**	**34**	**470**

Note: Numbers refer to number of grafts examined.

thrombotic event is related to the use of heparin. There is considerable evidence to show that thrombin is still generated during the bypass period, despite apparently adequate anticoagulation. Clinical experience suggests that the major actions of heparin to prevent thrombosis during open heart surgery occur via its actions on antithrombin III and may also be related to its action on the endothelium. By stimulating the release of the tissue factor pathway inhibitor, a serpin that inhibits both factor Xa and the tissue factor/VIIa complex, heparin will inhibit coagulation at a local level rather than through its effect on antithrombin III.[92]

Patients in whom thrombotic episodes were reported and who were also receiving aprotinin may have received less heparin than did patients in the placebo groups. This may have been a result of insufficient information being given to the investigators with regard to the need for additional doses of heparin to maintain adequate anticoagulation. In the past 12 months, considerable literature on this topic has suggested that monitoring the effects of heparin in the presence of aprotinin is problematic. In the early studies from Europe, the activator used to initiate coagulation was the diatomaceous earth celite. In early studies, aprotinin used in a high-dose regimen was shown to interfere with the activation of coagulation produced by this agent.[3] More recent studies have suggested that if kaolin is used as the activator, it absorbs the aprotinin and prevents its additional anticoagulant activity.[93] This has led to claims that kaolin-activated ACT is unaffected by aprotinin therapy.[94–97]

This conclusion may not be entirely justified for three reasons. First, aprotinin will prolong the activated partial thromboplastin time and have additive/synergistic effects with heparin, regardless of which of three standard activators (celite, kaolin, or ellegic acid) is used.[98] Second, there is increasing evidence that the activated coagulation time does not correlate with the effect of heparin or the degree of anticoagulation (inhibition of factor Xa) achieved.[3, 18, 99] Third, studies suggesting the superiority or improved reliability of the kaolin-activated ACT have been performed with low concentrations of aprotinin in spiked blood samples. Higher concentrations of aprotinin (300–600 KIU/mL), as found routinely when the high-dose regimen was used[3] and, also, after administration of a low- or 'half-dose' regimen,[100, 101] may still prolong the ACT with this activator. For example, a 50% reduction in activation of Factor XII after stimulation with kaolin occurs at concentrations of aprotinin of 330 KIU/mL.[102] This was the mean plasma concentration reported during bypass using a 'half-dose' regimen.[100, 101] To ensure that an adequate dose of heparin has been administered, it appears prudent to maintain the ACT at 750 seconds, regardless of the activator used, as recommended in earlier studies of the use of high-dose aprotinin.[2, 3, 103]

The lysine analogues have no apparent action on the control of anticoagulation. One study has suggested that clot formation is more easily seen with the use of epsilon-amino caproic acid, despite a reduction in the use of clotting factors.[104] There are no studies of the effects of the lysine analogues on graft patency or the incidence of myocardial ischemia.

RENAL DYSFUNCTION

The elimination of aprotinin from the circulation is, in part, a result of its absorption and re-uptake into the brush border of the renal tubule.[105] It has been suggested, therefore, that a high dose of aprotinin may overload the system, thereby leading to reduced tubular function and, thus, a degree of dysfunction of the kidney.[106]

The situation, as in all such discussions, is far from simple. We also know that renal function is altered by a large number of other neural and hormonal control mechanisms. In the latter category, the compounds kallikrein and natriuretic peptides (ANP) are primary players. In addition, a number of secondary controller mechanisms work through this system based on renin-aldosterone. In turn, the renin-aldosterone system is controlled by the angiotensin-converting enzyme (ACE) in the lung.

In this complex system, kallikrein and renin are serine proteases and are inhibited by high concentrations of aprotinin.[107–109] In contrast, the aminopeptidase activity in the kidney is augmented in the presence of low concentrations of aprotinin but is inhibited at high concentrations.[110] During bypass, the lungs are excluded from the circulation for a period; therefore, there is a diminution in ACE activity. In contrast to these events that tend to reduce concentrations of control hormones, the peptidase that destroys ANP is also inhibited by aprotinin. Indeed, aprotinin is added to all assay tubes in which these transient controlling peptides are measured to allow the assay to reflect true concentrations. This would suggest that concentrations of ANP in the plasma might be increased in the presence of aprotinin therapy. This potential for an increase in the concentration of active ANP may suggest that renal output could be improved during administration of aprotinin. This suggestion is supported by data showing that infusion of active ANP and its fragment is associated with improved renal function and outcome after complex heart surgery.

These dichotomous actions may explain some of the data related to renal function associated with cardiac surgery and the use of high-dose aprotinin therapy. Early studies concentrated on the first 48 hours after open heart surgery to investigate renal function. Studies in patients undergoing primary coronary artery bypass graft surgery showed that the excretion of sodium and free water was increased in the immediate postoperative period and in the period in the ICU.[111] Our own study and other early studies also suggested that the use of aprotinin was associated with an increase in the output of urine in the first 24 hours after surgery.[21] In patients undergoing reoperation surgery, renal function was assessed in the early postoperative period by measuring the creatinine clearance. In this study from the Cleveland Clinic Foundation, patients receiving infusions of placebo had a creatinine clearance of approximately 110 mL/min, and those in the high-dose aprotinin group had a clearance of approximately 132 mL/min.[32] This change did not achieve statistical significance; however, there obviously was no deleterious effect of aprotinin on creatinine clearance during this period.

In contrast to these studies of the early period, recent studies have investigated alterations in renal function that have occurred in the later period after cardiac surgery—up to approximately 7 days after the surgery had finished. The results of these studies have suggested that there is a significant difference in aspects related to renal function between those patients receiving aprotinin therapy and those in the placebo or controlled group. It seems appropriate to cite three studies in particular. The first is from a multicenter study performed in North America in patients having both primary and reoperation cardiac revascularization.[112] In these patients, there was a significant increase in the plasma concentration of creatinine on the fifth postoperative day compared with patients in the placebo group. Although the increase was significant statistically, the actual values were still within the laboratories' normal range for these patients. On further analysis of the data, it was also found that in those patients who had the worst renal function before their surgery, as shown by preoperative creatinine concentrations, there was no increased deleterious action of aprotinin. Also, there was no increase in the need for dialysis or renal support in the aprotinin-treated patients, despite this significant increase in later days' creatinine concentration.

The second study suggesting effects of high-dose aprotinin in later periods comes from a report of the use of aprotinin in patients undergoing surgery for the insertion of a left ventricular assist device (Heartmate, TCI instruments).[28] Goldstein and colleagues reported their results of using aprotinin therapy in 42 patients having a left ventricular assist device inserted and compared these results with those in 100 patients who did not receive aprotinin for the same procedure. In this study, the authors showed that, on the third day after the operation, there was a highly significant difference between the plasma concentrations of creatinine in patients who had received aprotinin compared with such concentrations in non–aprotinin-treated patients. Despite this obvious adverse effect on this biochemical end point related to renal function, the authors not only showed that the aprotinin-treated patients required fewer blood products, as would have been anticipated, but they also, most intriguingly, had a significantly reduced mortality and morbidity. The effects of mortality and morbidity may have been related to the time course of the study and a 'learning curve' in relation to insertion of this particular assist device.

From the data presented, it is more difficult to understand that despite the highly significant increase in the creatinine concentration in the patients who received aprotinin therapy, there was no change in the concentrations of blood urea nitrogen (BUN). It is difficult to define a system whereby BUN is unchanged and creatinine concentration increases with a specific action of a nephrotoxic drug. This might imply that the increase in the creatinine level is associated with some other action of the aprotinin therapy—particularly in relation to its effect on tissue and muscle metabolism. Since the early 1960s, it has been well known that aprotinin has significant actions to modify the process of muscle function and, in particular, intermediate metabolism. Indeed, one of the earliest studies looking at the effects of aprotinin in patients undergoing hip surgery was specifically aimed at reducing the amount of lactic acid produced during the operative procedure in these patients.[113] Other studies in patients undergoing vascular surgery showed that there was reduced release of acid after reperfusion of the lower torso.[114] The potential role of aprotinin in reducing reperfusion injury has recently been reviewed.[75]

The third—and most recent—study suggesting that aprotinin has an action on the kidney in the latter part of the postoperative period comes from an investigation of the excretion of protein from the kidney in the first 5 days after surgery.[115] These studies showed that the processes of cardiopulmonary bypass and heart surgery alone were sufficient to induce a mild but statistically significant increase in protein excretion in the days after surgery. In those patients receiving aprotinin therapy, the protein excretion was described as being greater. The increase did not achieve statistical significance, however, for the excretion of proteins filtered by the tubules or the glomeruli. Similarly, in this study there was no significant difference between the total protein and albumin fractions of the excreted protein fractions.

The biological relevance of these latter three studies needs to be the subject of greater research and thought. It may be true that aprotinin is shown to be a mild nephrotoxic agent. However, the biological relevance of this is totally unclear. In many centers in North America, patients are being discharged on the fifth postoperative day. The study by Feindt and colleagues showed that one aspect of renal function is abnormal at this time. In a similar way, it is also true that respiratory function still shows abnormalities when using sensitive tests up to the seventh day after the operation. At this time, however, the patients are usually ambulatory and self-caring, and they are usually out of the hospital.

What is probably required is carefully documented (without hysteria or prejudice) case reports suggesting where there may be additive reasons why the use of high-dose aprotinin will produce a severe and biologically relevant impairment of renal function. At this time, the only such report is one by Sundt and colleagues from St Louis, who reported an uncontrolled group of patients who were having aortic surgery with hypothermic arrest.[116] They noted that more patients in this group appeared to have renal failure and to have evidence of a coagulopathy, which appeared to be associated with an increased mortality. This report can be harshly criticized on a number of levels; however, in my opinion, it was a simple attempt to bring to the attention of the clinical and scientific community one group's experience—one that they thought might warrant further examination. It is unfortunate that instead of stimulating clinicians to provide controlled studies, this report produced an hysterical response within North America, suggesting that aprotinin may kill all patients who have deep hypothermic circulatory arrest. This is obviously untrue, because this procedure has been used within Europe on many occasions and is still routinely used for various surgeries at my institute, without there being any obvious deleterious effect to the patient or to his/her renal function. Because of the perceived beneficial effects of high-dose aprotinin in patients having complex surgery with hypothermic arrest as used in Europe, most centers will not consider including a placebo group in any study. Therefore, the question of the use of aprotinin in such procedures must still be based on prejudice and not on scientific fact.

HYPERSENSITIVITY RESPONSES

The incidence and severity of hypersensitivity responses are of critical importance when considering the use of high-dose aprotinin therapy, because they may influence the clinician and the use of the compound in first-time operative procedures.

Aprotinin is a naturally occurring compound that is usually obtained from bovine lung. However, approximately 5% of the world's supply is obtained from porcine gut. In this regard, this represents the exact reverse of the production of heparin. Both aprotinin and heparin are obtained from the mast cell, where they are found together. The mast cell is the only site in the body where heparin and aprotinin are routinely found. The precise reason for heparin and aprotinin being found in mast cells remains to be elucidated. In vivo, heparin is an anti-inflammatory agent as opposed to an anticoagulant. Presumably, this has some bearing on the finding of these two substances at the same site.

In the recent literature, there are three reports of large numbers of patients being treated with high doses of aprotinin; these suggest that the incidence of hypersensitivity responses is in the range of 0.3% to 0.6% of administrations.[70, 117, 118] These responses have included minor skin rashes, minor changes in cardiovascular function, and the continuing spectrum up to true anaphylactic reactions. In this regard, the incidence of hypersensitivity responses is approximately the same as that found with a number of other agents used during cardiac surgery, including muscle relaxants[119] and plasma expanders.[120]

The major problem to be discussed is the incidence of severe reactions to the agent. In the recent literature, four reports have suggested severe cardiovascular collapse when the agent was given.[121–124] It is worthwhile considering each of these anecdotal reports to discover whether the patient had an anaphylactic reaction. It is obvious that for a patient to have a true anaphylactic reaction, he/she must have an IgE antibody to the agent. This is as defined by the Gell and Coombes classification of reactions. The presence of such an antibody can usually be demonstrated by previous skin testing of the agent with a small intradermal injection. At present, my routine practice is to perform such a test before following the manufacturer's instructions to give a small (1-mL) IV test dose of the agent with appropriate patient monitoring. In contrast to this approach, in three of the four patients who were reported to have had a major cardiovascular collapse during administration of aprotinin, this collapse was said to have occurred after the infusion of 200 mL, 75 mL, and 50 mL, respectively, of the solution.[121, 122, 124] In the first and second cases, the manufacturer's instructions clearly were not followed, as these patients received 4 and 1.5 vials of a substance, respectively, intravenously, before any evidence of a cardiovascular collapse. It is well recognized in the literature from the early 1960s that a rapid infusion of aprotinin is associated with a small decrease in blood pressure in approximately 20% of patients.[9] The rapid infusion of large volumes of solution into patients who have critical coronary stenosis and ischemic myocardium cannot be condoned.

The last[123] of these four reports and subsequent studies from centers within Germany[125] have confirmed that there is a definite chance of a true anaphylactic reaction occurring after a second exposure to aprotinin. Most of these cases have occurred when the second administration is within six months of the first. The most recent report from Germany surveyed 248 patients who had definitely received aprotinin on a previous occasion for their cardiac surgery. In this group, the incidence of a true reaction was estimated to be 2.5%. This seems to be a reasonable figure for the incidence of anaphylaxis after a guaranteed reexposure to the drug within a 6-month time frame.

If previous exposure during this period is known, it is suggested that the patient have, in the first instance, an intradermal prick test using aprotinin solution. If this does not produce a wheel-and-flare response, then it is probably safe to continue administering the test dose. In many institutions, the process has now been further modified. The test dose of aprotinin solution is not administered, and, therefore, administration of the loading dose is not begun until the patient is in the operating room and has been draped and the sternotomy has been performed. The rationale for this approach is that if there is a severe reaction during the test dose or loading dose, then heparin can be administered and bypass can be initiated more rapidly. In addition, certain centers advocate the use of histamine receptor blockade with both H1- and H2-blockers before the administration of the aprotinin test dose. Whether this is of any benefit in preventing or reducing the severity of reaction is currently unknown.

REFERENCES

1. Davis R, Whittington R: Aprotinin: A review of its pharmacology and therapeutic efficacy in reducing blood loss associated with cardiac surgery. *Drugs* 49:954–983, 1995.
2. Royston D: The serine antiprotease aprotinin (Trasylol): A novel approach to reducing postoperative bleeding. *Blood Coagul Fibrinolysis* 1:55–69, 1990.
3. Royston D: High-dose aprotinin therapy: A review of the first five years' experience. *J Cardiothorac Vasc Anesth* 6:76–100, 1992.

4. Beecher A, Todd D: A study of the deaths associated with anesthesia and surgery based on a study of 59,548 anesthesias in 10 institutions, 1948–1952 inclusive. *Ann Surg* 140:2–35, 1954.
5. Viljoen JF, Estafanous FG, Kellner GA: Propranolol and cardiac surgery. *J Thorac Cardiovasc Surg* 64:826–830, 1972.
6. Bunker J: *The National Halothane Study: A Study of the Possible Association Between Halothane Anesthesia and Hepatic Necrosis.* 1969, National Institutes of Health, Bethesda, Maryland.
7. Fears. *Fibrinolysis* In press, 1992.
8. Dietrich W, Spannagl M, Jochum M, et al: Influence of high-dose aprotinin treatment on blood loss and coagulation patterns in patients undergoing myocardial revascularization [see comments]. *Anesthesiology* 73:1119–1126, 1990.
9. Fritz H, Wunderer G: Biochemistry and applications of aprotinin, the kallikrein inhibitor from bovine organs. *Arzneimittelforschung* 33:479–494, 1983.
10. Verstraete M: Clinical application of inhibitors of fibrinolysis. *Drugs* 29:236–261, 1983.
11. Dietrich W: Reduced thrombin formation during cardiopulmonary bypass: Is there a benefit of the additional anticoagulant action of aprotinin? *J Cardiovasc Pharmacol* 27:S50–S57, 1996.
12. Dietrich W, Spannagl M, Dooijewaard G, et al: Protection of single chain urokinase plasminogen activator (SCUPA) by aprotinin in patients undergoing cardio-pulmonary bypass (CPB) is due to contact phase inhibition. *Anesthesiology* 81:A87, 1994.
13. Schleef RR, Bevilacqua MP, Sawdey M, et al: Cytokine activation of vascular endothelium: Effects on tissue-type plasminogen activator and type 1 plasminogen activator inhibitor. *J Biol Chem* 263:5797–5803, 1988.
14. van Hinsbergh VW: Regulation of the synthesis and secretion of plasminogen activators by endothelial cells. *Haemostasis* 18:307–327, 1988.
15. Ruggeroli A, Carruthers R, Pohorecki R, et al: Cardiopulmonary bypass-induced inflammation: Steroids v aprotinin (Abstract). *Anesthesiology* 83:A83, 1995.
16. Whitten C, Latson T, Allison P, et al: Does aprotinin inhibit cardiopulmonary bypass induced inflammation? *Anesthesiology* 77:A266, 1992.
17. Kluft C, Dooijewaard G, Emeis JJ: Role of the contact system in fibrinolysis. *Semin Thromb Hemost* 13:50–68, 1987.
18. Feindt P, Volkmer I, Seyfert U, et al: Activated clotting time, anticoagulation, use of heparin, and thrombin activation during extracorporeal circulation: Changes under aprotinin therapy. *Thorac Cardiovasc Surg* 41:9–15, 1993.
19. Lu H, Soria C, Commin PL, et al: Hemostasis in patients undergoing extracorporeal circulation: The effect of aprotinin (Trasylol). *Thromb Haemost* 66:633–637, 1991.

20. Lu H, Du Buit C, Soria J, et al: Postoperative hemostasis and fibrinolysis in patients undergoing cardiopulmonary bypass with or without aprotinin therapy. *Thromb Haemost* 72:438–443, 1994.
21. Bidstrup BP, Royston D, Sapsford RN, et al: Reduction in blood loss and blood use after cardiopulmonary bypass with high dose aprotinin (Trasylol). *J Thorac Cardiovasc Surg* 97:364–372, 1989.
22. Havel M, Owen AN, Simon P, et al: Decreasing use of donated blood and reduction of bleeding after orthotopic heart transplantation by use of aprotinin. *J Heart Lung Transplant* 11:348–349, 1992.
23. Jaquiss RD, Huddleston CB, Spray TL: Use of aprotinin in pediatric lung transplantation. *J Heart Lung Transplant* 14:302–307, 1995.
24. Kesten S, de Hoyas A, Chaparro C, et al: Aprotinin reduces blood loss in lung transplant recipients. *Ann Thorac Surg* 59:877–879, 1995.
25. Peterson KL, DeCampli WM, Feeley TW, et al: Blood loss and transfusion requirements in cystic fibrosis patients undergoing heart-lung or lung transplantation. *J Cardiothorac Vasc Anesth* 9:59–62, 1995.
26. Royston D: Aprotinin therapy in heart and heart-lung transplantation. *J Heart Lung Transplant* 12:S19–S25, 1993.
27. Propst JW, Siegel LC, Feeley TW: Effect of aprotinin on transfusion requirements during repeat sternotomy for cardiac transplantation surgery. *Transplant Proc* 26:3719–3721, 1994.
28. Goldstein D, Selmonridge J, Chen J, et al: Use of aprotinin in LVAD recipients reduces blood loss, blood use and perioperative mortality. *Ann Thorac Surg* 59:1063–1068, 1995.
29. Brunel F, Mira JP, Belghith M, et al: Effects of aprotinin on hemorrhagic complications in ARDS patients during prolonged extracorporeal CO2 removal. *Intensive Care Med* 18:364–367, 1992.
30. Takahama T, Kanai F, Hiraishi M, et al: Comparative study of anticoagulation therapy with an LVAD system. *ASAIO Trans* 33:227–234, 1987.
31. Bidstrup B, Royston D, McGuiness C, et al: Aprotinin in aspirin-pretreated patients. *Perfusion* 5:77–81, 1990.
32. Cosgrove DM III, Heric B, Lytle BW, et al: Aprotinin therapy for reoperative myocardial revascularization: A placebo-controlled study [see comments]. *Ann Thorac Surg* 54:1031–1036, 1992.
33. Murkin J, Lux J, Shannon N, et al: Aprotinin significantly decreases bleeding and transfusion requirements in patients receiving aspirin and undergoing cardiac operations. *J Thorac Cardiovasc Surg* 107:554–561, 1994.
34. Deviri E, Izhar U, Drenger B, et al: Aprotinin treatment during open heart operation in a patient with severe thrombocytopenia [letter]. *Ann Thorac Surg* 54:1018–1019, 1992.
35. Akhtar TM, Goodchild CS, Boylan MK: Reversal of streptokinase-induced bleeding with aprotinin for emergency cardiac surgery. *Anaesthesia* 47:226–228, 1992.
36. Efstratiadis T, Munsch C, Crossman D, et al: Aprotinin used in emer-

gency coronary operation after streptokinase treatment [see comments]. *Ann Thorac Surg* 52:1320–1321, 1991.

37. van-Doorn CA, Munsch CM, Cowan JC: Cardiac rupture after thrombolytic therapy: The use of aprotinin to reduce blood loss after surgical repair. *Br Heart J* 67:504–505, 1992.
38. Dietrich W, Dilthey G, Spannagl M, et al: Warfarin pretreatment does not lead to increased bleeding tendency during cardiac surgery. *J Cardiothorac Vasc Anesth* 9:250–254, 1995.
39. Taenaka N, Shimada Y, Hirata T, et al: New approach to regional anticoagulation in hemodialysis using gabexate mesilate (FOY). *Crit Care Med* 10:773–775, 1982.
40. Taenaka N, Terada N, Takahashi H, et al: Hemodialysis using gabexate mesilate (FOY) in patients with a high bleeding risk. *Crit Care Med* 14:481–483, 1986.
41. Thompson J, Roath S, Francis J, et al: Aprotinin in peripheral vascular surgery. *Lancet* 335:911, 1990.
42. Lord RA, Roath OS, Thompson JF, et al: Effect of aprotinin on neutrophil function after major vascular surgery. *Br J Surg* 79:517–521, 1992.
43. Bechstein WO, Riess H, Blumhardt G, et al: Aprotinin in orthotopic liver transplantation. *Semin Thromb Hemost* 19:262–267, 1993.
44. Gerlach H, Rossaint R, Slama K, et al: No requirement for cryoprecipitate or platelet transfusion during liver transplantation. *Transplant Proc* 25:1813–1816, 1993.
45. Mallett S, Rolles K, Cox D, et al: Intraoperative use of aprotinin (Trasylol) in orthotopic liver transplantation. *Transplant Proc* 23:1931–1932, 1991.
46. Patrassi GM, Viero M, Sartori MT, et al: Aprotinin efficacy on intraoperative bleeding and transfusion requirements in orthotopic liver transplantation. *Transfusion* 34:507–511, 1994.
47. Smith O, Hazlehurst G, Brozovic B, et al: Impact of aprotinin on blood transfusion requirements in liver transplantation. *Transfus Med* 3:97–102, 1993.
48. Janssens M, Joris J, David JL, et al: High-dose aprotinin reduces blood loss in patients undergoing total hip replacement surgery [see comments]. *Anesthesiology* 80:23–29, 1994.
49. Murkin JM, Shannon NA, Bourne RB, et al: Aprotinin decreases blood loss in patients undergoing revision or bilateral total hip arthroplasty. *Anesth Analg* 80:343–348, 1995.
50. Giromini D, Tzonos T: Local use of aprotinin in neurosurgical operations for the prevention of hyperfibrinolytic hemorrhage. *Fortschr Med* 99:1153–1156, 1981.
51. Palmer JD, Francis DA, Roath OS, et al: Hyperfibrinolysis during intracranial surgery: Effect of high dose aprotinin. *J Neurol Neurosurg Psychiatry* 58:104–106, 1995.
52. Tzonos T, Giromini D: Aprotinin for intraoperative haemostasis. *Neurosurg Rev* 4:193–194, 1981.
53. Sher G: Trasylol in the management of abruptio placentae with con-

sumption coagulopathy and uterine inertia. *J Reprod Med* 25:113–118, 1980.

54. Sher G, Statland BE: Abruptio placentae with coagulopathy: A rational basis for management. *Clin Obstet Gynecol* 28:15–23, 1985.
55. Astedt B: Clinical pharmacology of tranexamic acid. *Scand J Gastroenterol Suppl* 137:22–25, 1987.
56. Horrow J: Management of coagulation and bleeding disorders, in Kaplan J (ed): *Cardiac Anesthesia.* Philadelphia, PA, W.B. Saunders and Co., 1993, pp 951–994.
57. de Bono D, Pringle S, Underwood I: Differential effects of aprotinin and tranexamic acid on cerebral bleeding and cutaneous bleeding time during rt-PA infusion. *Thromb Res* 61:159–163, 1991.
58. Royston D: Blood-sparing drugs: Aprotinin, tranexamic acid, and epsilon-aminocaproic acid. *Int Anesthesiol Clin* 33:155–179, 1995.
59. Tsementzis SA, Honan WP, Nightingale S, et al: Fibrinolytic activity after subarachnoid haemorrhage and the effect of tranexamic acid. *Acta Neurochir Wien* 103:116–121, 1990.
60. Tsementzis SA, Hitchcock ER, Meyer CH: Benefits and risks of antifibrinolytic therapy in the management of ruptured intracranial aneurysms: A double-blind placebo-controlled study. *Acta Neurochir Wien* 102:1–10, 1990.
61. Davies D, Howell DA: Tranexamic acid and arterial thrombosis [letter]. *Lancet* 1:49, 1977.
62. Fodstad H, Liliequist B: Spontaneous thrombosis of ruptured intracranial aneurysms during treatment with tranexamic acid (AMCA): Report of three cases. *Acta Neurochir Wien* 49:129–144, 1979.
63. Hoffman EP, Koo AH: Cerebral thrombosis associated with Amicar therapy. *Radiology* 131:687–689, 1979.
64. Haley E Jr., Torner JC, Kassell NF: Antifibrinolytic therapy and cerebral vasospasm. *Neurosurg Clin North Am* 1:349–356, 1990.
65. Anon: Protease inhibitors for delayed cerebral ischemia after subarachnoid haemorrhage? [editorial]. *Lancet* 339:1199–2000, 1992.
66. Yanamoto H, Kikuchi H, Sato M, et al: Therapeutic trial of cerebral vasospasm with the serine protease inhibitor, FUT-175, administered in the acute stage after subarachnoid hemorrhage. *Neurosurgery* 30:358–363, 1992.
67. Yanamoto H, Kikuchi H, Okamoto S, et al: Preventive effects of synthetic serine protease inhibitor, FUT-175, on cerebral vasospasm in rabbits. *Neurosurgery* 30:351–356, 1992.
68. Guidetti B, Spallone A: The role of antifibrinolytic therapy in the preoperative management of recently ruptured intracranial aneurysms. *Surg Neurol* 15:239–248, 1981.
69. Kamiya T, Katayama Y, Kashiwagi F, et al: The role of bradykinin in mediating ischaemic brain edema in rats. *Stroke* 24:571–576, 1993.
70. Bidstrup BP, Harrison J, Royston D, et al: Aprotinin therapy in cardiac operations: A report on use in 41 cardiac centers in the United Kingdom. *Ann Thorac Surg* 55:971–976, 1993.

71. Lytle BW, Loop FD, Cosgrove DM, et al: Fifteen hundred coronary reoperations: Results and determinants of early and late survival. *J Thorac Cardiovasc Surg* 93:847–859, 1987.
72. Jones E, Weintraub W, Craver J: Coronary bypass surgery: Is the operation different today? *J Thorac Cardiovasc Surg* 101:108–115, 1991.
73. Dietrich W, Barankay A, Niekau E, et al: High dose aprotinin in cardiac surgery: Old drug-new aspects of homologous blood requirement, in Birnbaum D, Hoffmeister H (ed): *Blood Saving in Open Heart Surgery.* Stuttgart–New York, Schattauer, 1990, pp 76–82.
74. Levy J, Pifarre R, Schaff H, et al: A multicenter double-blind, placebo-controlled trial of aprotinin for reducing blood loss and the requirement for donor-blood transfusion in patients having repeat coronary artery bypass grafting. *Circulation* 92:2236–2244, 1995.
75. Royston D: Preventing the inflammatory response to open-heart surgery: The role of aprotinin and other protease inhibitors. *Int J Cardiol* 1996. In press.
76. Royston D: Serine protease inhibition prevents both cellular and humoral responses to cardiopulmonary bypass. *J Cardiovasc Pharmacol* 27:S42–S49, 1996.
77. Fish KJ, Sarnquist FH, van Steennis C, et al: A prospective, randomized study of the effects of prostacyclin on platelets and blood loss during coronary bypass operations. *J Thorac Cardiovasc Surg* 91:436–442, 1986.
78. Moorehead M, Westernguard J, Bull B: Platelet involvement in the activated coagulation time of heparinized blood. *Anesth Analg* 63:394–398, 1984.
79. Bode AP, Castellani WJ, Hodges ED, et al: The effect of lysed platelets on neutralization of heparin in vitro with protamine as measured by the activated coagulation time (ACT) [published erratum appears in *Thromb Haemost* 66(6):746, Dec 2 1991]. *Thromb Haemost* 66:213–217, 1991.
80. Despotis G, Joist J, Hogue C, et al: The effect of higher heparin concentrations on preservation of hemostasis in cardiac surgical patients [abstract]. *Anesthesiology* 83:A91, 1995.
81. Spannagl M, Dietrich W, Beck A, et al: High dose aprotinin reduces prothrombin and fibrinogen conversion in patients undergoing extracorporeal circulation for myocardial revascularization [letter]. *Thromb Haemost* 72:159–160, 1994.
82. Harker LA: Bleeding after cardiopulmonary bypass [editorial]. *N Engl J Med* 314:1446–1448, 1986.
83. Hamm CW, Reimers J, Ischinger T, et al: A randomized study of coronary angioplasty compared with bypass surgery in patients with symptomatic multivessel coronary disease: German Angioplasty Bypass Surgery Investigation (GABI) [see comments]. *N Engl J Med* 331:1037–1043, 1994.
84. King SBr, Lembo NJ, Weintraub WS, et al: A randomized trial comparing coronary angioplasty with coronary bypass surgery: Emory An-

gioplasty versus Surgery Trial (EAST) [see comments]. *N Engl J Med* 331:1044–1050, 1994.
85. van der Meer J, Hillege HL, van Gilst WH, et al: A comparison of internal mammary artery and saphenous vein grafts after coronary artery bypass surgery: No difference in 1-year occlusion rates and clinical outcome. CABADAS Research Group of the Interuniversity Cardiology Institute of The Netherlands. *Circulation* 90:2367–2374, 1994.
86. Bidstrup BP, Underwood SR, Sapsford RN, et al: Effect of aprotinin (Trasylol) on aorta-coronary bypass graft patency. *J Thorac Cardiovasc Surg* 105:147–152, 1993.
87. Havel M, Grabenwoger F, Schneider J, et al: Aprotinin does not decrease early graft patency after coronary artery bypass grafting despite reducing postoperative bleeding and use of donated blood. *J Thorac Cardiovasc Surg* 107:807–810, 1994.
88. Lass M, Welz A, Kochs M, et al: Aprotinin in elective primary bypass surgery: Graft patency and clinical efficacy. *Eur J Cardiothorac Surg* 9:206–210, 1995.
89. Lemmer J Jr, Stanford W, Bonney SL, et al: Aprotinin for coronary bypass operations: efficacy, safety, and influence on early saphenous vein graft patency: A multicenter, randomized, double-blind, placebo-controlled study. *J Thorac Cardiovasc Surg* 107:543–551, 1994.
90. Laub GW, Riebman JB, Chen C, et al: The impact of aprotinin on coronary artery bypass graft patency. *Chest* 106:1370–1375, 1994.
91. Ollivier J, EPPAC plg: Étude de la perméabilité des pontages aorto-coronaires à 6 mois: Étude multicentrique française. *Arch Mal Coeur* 84:53–542, 1991.
92. Abildgaard U: Heparin/low molecular weight heparin and tissue factor pathway inhibitor. *Haemostasis* 1:103–106, 1993.
93. Dietrich W, Jochum M: Effect of celite and kaolin on activated clotting time in the presence of aprotinin: Activated clotting time is reduced by binding of aprotinin to kaolin. *J Thorac Cardiovasc Surg* 109:177–178, 1995.
94. Farooqi N, De-Hert S, Vlaeminck R, et al: Effects of low doses of aprotinin on clotting times activated with celite and kaolin. *Acta Anaesthesiol Belg* 44:87–92, 1993.
95. Feindt P, Seyfert UT, Volkmer I, et al: Celite and kaolin produce differing activated clotting times during cardiopulmonary bypass under aprotinin therapy. *Thorac Cardiovasc Surg* 42:218–221, 1994.
96. Wendel HP, Heller W, Gallimore MJ, et al: The prolonged activated clotting time (ACT) with aprotinin depends on the type of activator used for measurement. *Blood Coagul Fibrinolysis* 4:41–45, 1993.
97. Wang JS, Lin CY, Hung WT, et al: Monitoring of heparin-induced anticoagulation with kaolin-activated clotting time in cardiac surgical patients treated with aprotinin. *Anesthesiology* 77:1080–1084, 1992.
98. Francis JL, Howard C: The effect of aprotinin on the response of the activated partial thromboplastin time (APTT) to heparin. *Blood Coagul Fibrinolysis* 4:35–40, 1993.

99. Despotis GJ, Joist JH, Joiner Maier D, et al: Effect of aprotinin on activated clotting time, whole blood and plasma heparin measurements. *Ann Thorac Surg* 59:106–111, 1995.
100. Liu B, Belboul A, Radberg G, et al: Effect of reduced aprotinin dosage on blood loss and use of blood products in patients undergoing cardiopulmonary bypass. *Scand J Thorac Cardiovasc Surg* 27:149–155, 1993.
101. Liu B, Tengborn L, Larson G, et al: Half-dose aprotinin preserves hemostatic function in patients undergoing bypass operations. *Ann Thorac Surg* 59:1534–1540, 1995.
102. Laurel MT, Ratnoff OD, Everson B: Inhibition of the activation of Hageman factor (factor XII) by aprotinin (Trasylol). *J Lab Clin Med* 119:580–585, 1992.
103. Hunt BJ, Segal H, Yacoub M: Aprotinin and heparin monitoring during cardiopulmonary bypass. *Circulation* 86:II410–II412, 1992.
104. Arom KV, Emery RW: Decreased postoperative drainage with addition of epsilon-aminocaproic acid before cardiopulmonary bypass. *Ann Thorac Surg* 57:1108–1112, 1994.
105. Tenstad O, Williamson HE, Clausen G, et al: Glomerular filtration and tubular absorption of the basic polypeptide aprotinin. *Acta Physiol Scand* 152:33–50, 1994.
106. Westaby S: Aprotinin in perspective. *Ann Thorac Surg* 55:1033–1041, 1993.
107. Beierwaltes WH, Prada J, Carretero OA: Effect of glandular kallikrein on renin release in isolated rat glomeruli. *Hypertension* 7:27–31, 1985.
108. Madeddu P, Oppes M, Soro A, et al: The effects of aprotinin, a kallikrein inhibitor, on renin release and urinary sodium excretion in mild essential hypertensives. *J Hypertens* 5:581–586, 1987.
109. Sealey JE, Overlack A, Laragh JH, et al: Effect of captopril and aprotinin on inactive renin. *J Clin Endocrinol Metab* 53:626–630, 1981.
110. Scherberich JE, Mondorf W: Effect of a proteinase inhibitor, aprotinin, on brush border membrane associated aminopeptidase of human kidney cortex. *Arzneimittelforschung* 30:487–491, 1980.
111. Blauhut B, Gross C, Necek S, et al: Effects of high-dose aprotinin on blood loss, platelet function, fibrinolysis, complement, and renal function after cardiopulmonary bypass. *J Thorac Cardiovasc Surg* 101:958–967, 1991.
112. Lemmer JH Jr, Stanford W, Bonney SL, et al: Aprotinin for coronary artery bypass grafting: effect on postoperative renal function. *Ann Thorac Surg* 59:132–136, 1995.
113. Haas S, Ketterl R, Stemberger A, et al: The effect of aprotinin on platelet function, blood coagulation and blood lactate level in total hip replacement: A double blind clinical trial. *Adv Exp Med Biol* 167:287–297, 1984.
114. Horl M, Sperling M, Herzog I, et al: Effect of aprotinin on metabolic changes in blood following aortofemoral bypass operation. *Eur Surg Res* 17:186–196, 1985.

115. Feindt P, Walcher S, Volkmer I, et al: Effects of high-dose aprotinin on renal function in aortocoronary bypass grafting. *Ann Thorac Surg* 60:1076–1080, 1995.
116. Sundt T, Kouchoukos NT, Saffitz JE, et al: Renal dysfunction and intravascular coagulation with aprotinin and hypothermic circulatory arrest. *Ann Thorac Surg* 55:1418–1424, 1993.
117. Dietrich W, Barankay A, Hahnel C, et al: High-dose aprotinin in cardiac surgery: Three years' experience in 1,784 patients. *J Cardiothorac Vasc Anesth* 6:324–327, 1992.
118. Paroli A, Antona C, Gerometta P, et al: The effect of 'high dose' aprotinin and other factors on bleeding and revisions for bleeding in adult coronary and valve operations: an analysis of 2190 patients during a five-year period (1987–1991). *Eur J Cardiothorac Surg* 9:77–82, 1995.
119. Levy JH: Anaphylactic/anaphylactoid reactions during cardiac surgery. *J Clin Anesth* 1:426–430, 1989.
120. Laxenaire MC, Charpentier C, Feldman L: [Anaphylactoid reactions to colloid plasma substitutes: incidence, risk factors, mechanisms: A French multicenter prospective study]. *Ann Fr Anesth Reanim* 13:301–310, 1994.
121. Dewachter P, Mouton C, Masson C, et al: Anaphylactic reaction to aprotinin during cardiac surgery [letter]. *Anaesthesia* 48:1110–1111, 1993.
122. Diefenbach C, Abel M, Limpers B, et al: Fatal anaphylactic shock after aprotinin reexposure in cardiac surgery. *Anesth Analg* 80:830–831, 1995.
123. Ceriana P, Maurelli M, Locateli A, et al: Anaphylactic reaction to aprotinin. *J Cardiothorac Vasc Anesth* 9:477–478, 1995.
124. Schulze K, Graeter T, Schaps D, et al: Severe anaphylactic shock due to repeated application of aprotinin in patients following intrathoracic aortic replacement. *Eur J Cardiothorac Surg* 7:495–496, 1993.
125. Dietrich W, Späth P, Ebell A, et al: Incidence of anaphylactic reactions to aprotinin-analysis of 248 re-exposures to aprotinin [abstract]. *Anesthesiology* 83:104A, 1995.

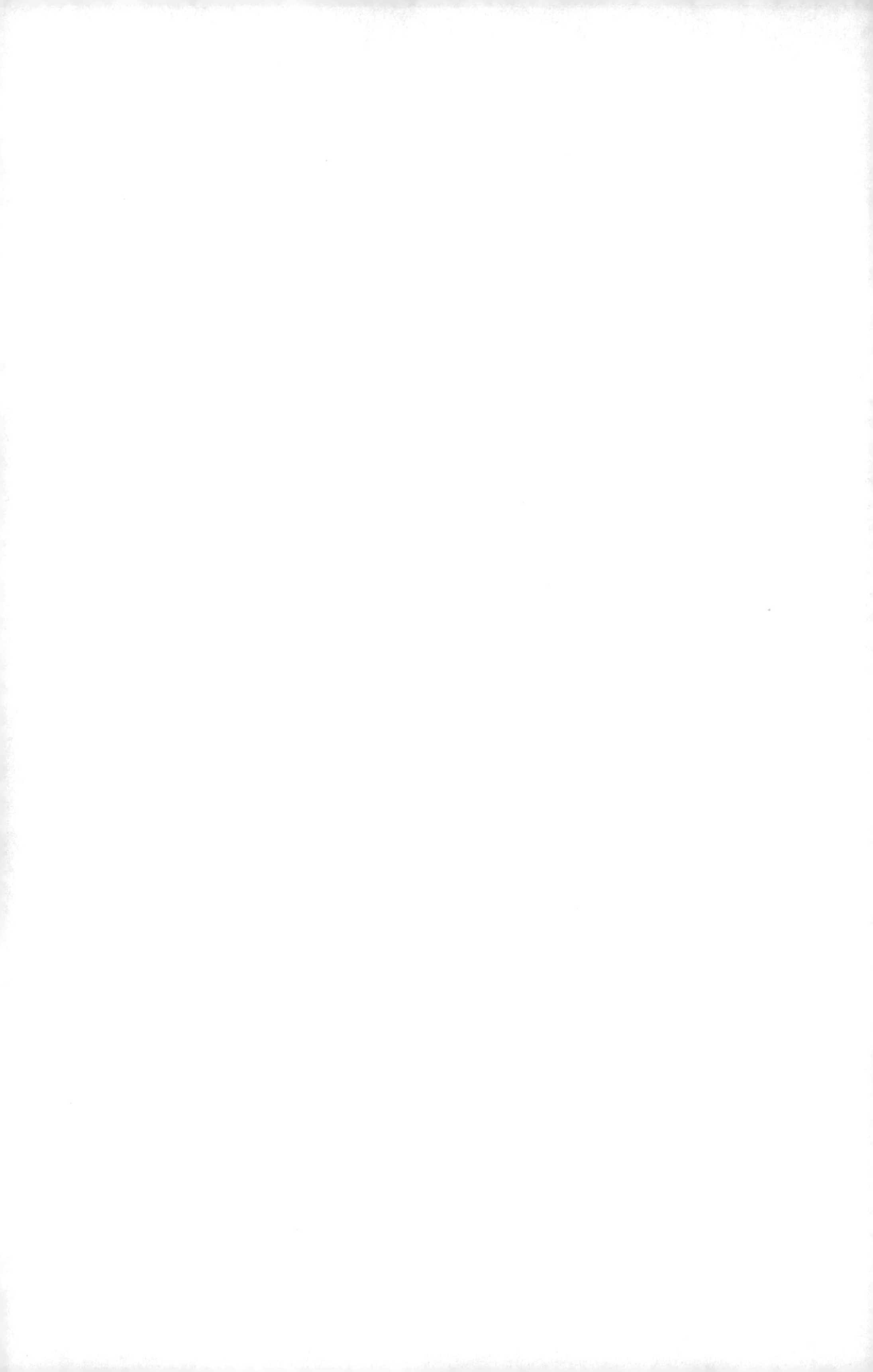

Vascular Biology of Coronary Artery Bypass Conduits: New Solutions to Old Problems?*

Alan J. Bryan, D.M., F.R.C.S.
Senior Lecturer, Bristol Heart Institute, University of Bristol, Bristol Royal Infirmary, England

Gianni D. Angelini, M.Ch., F.R.C.S.
British Heart Foundation Professor of Cardiac Surgery, Bristol Heart Institute, University of Bristol, Bristol Royal Infirmary, England

Coronary artery bypass grafting has been evolving for more than 30 years. More than 400,000 procedures are performed each year in the United States, with cardiac care accounting for as much as 25% of the total health care budget.[1] There are, therefore, overwhelming clinical and economic reasons to optimize early and late clinical outcome after coronary artery bypass grafting.

The early mortality associated with primary coronary bypass grafting remains approximately 2% to 4%, despite the increasing age of the patients and severity of disease being treated.[2] The main limitations to long-term outcome remain the problems of late vein graft failure and progresson of disease within the native coronary circulation. This inevitably leads to recurrent angina and need for reoperation in more than 10% of patients who underwent revascularization with saphenous vein grafts alone 10–12 years previously.[3] In the United States, 10% to 30% of coronary artery bypass grafting procedures are reoperations,[4, 5] whereas in the United Kingdom this proportion remains less than 5%.[2]

Surgeons have responded to these challenges in several ways. The improvements in both early and late survival conferred by the use of the pedicled left internal thoracic artery (ITA) graft to the left anterior descending coronary artery (LAD)[6–8] has made this a

*This work was supported by the British Heart Foundation and the Garfield Weston Trust.

© 1996, Mosby–Year Book, Inc.

routine part of the procedure whenever possible.[9] Further attempts to improve late outcome have been directed toward increased use of bilateral and complex ITA grafting and the evaluation of several alternative autologous arterial conduits.[10–12]

Despite these worthwhile strategies, the predominance of multiple grafting, the technical ease of use and availability, and the increasing need for repeat surgery mean that the saphenous vein continues to occupy a major role as a conduit for coronary artery bypass grafting. Indeed, recent calculations indicate that the saphenous vein continues to be used for more than 70% of grafts.[13] Research activity has therefore been directed toward a greater understanding of the degenerative changes that occur in vein grafts. Particular attention has been paid to the basic mechanisms of intimal vascular smooth muscle cell (VSMC) proliferation with superimposed late atheromatous change, as 50% of vein grafts become occluded within 10 years after the operation.[14] The application of molecular biological techniques and the development of in vitro cell and organ culture systems and in vivo animal models have provided a plethora of new information, not only about autocrine and paracrine influences on endothelial and VSMC function but also on the structure, function, and potential for modulation of vascular-cell genes.[15–18] Advances such as these offer enormous potential for the development of strategies to prevent intimal hyperplasia; however, effective and practical methods to achieve this goal in the clinical setting remain elusive.

PATHOPHYSIOLOGY OF GRAFT FAILURE

Autologous vein implanted into the arterial circulation has a characteristic sequence of adaptive pathologic changes that may lead ultimately to graft failure. Detailed knowledge of the changes that occur in saphenous vein grafts has come from serial angiographic studies of patients after coronary artery bypass grafting.[14, 19] These observations have been supplemented with studies of the cellular and morphologic changes of human pathologic specimens[20–23] and detailed time course experiments in comparable animal models.[24–26] Arterial grafts, because they are already adapted to the physiology of the arterial circulation, manifest few morphologic changes and predominantly alter their flow patterns and vasomotor responses to supply the different requirements of the coronary circulation (Fig 1).

At the time of implantation into the arterial circulation, the vein has inevitably been subjected to surgical preparation, which may result in vessel wall injury. Classification of vessel wall damage[27, 28] identifies a spectrum of injury, from type I (functional

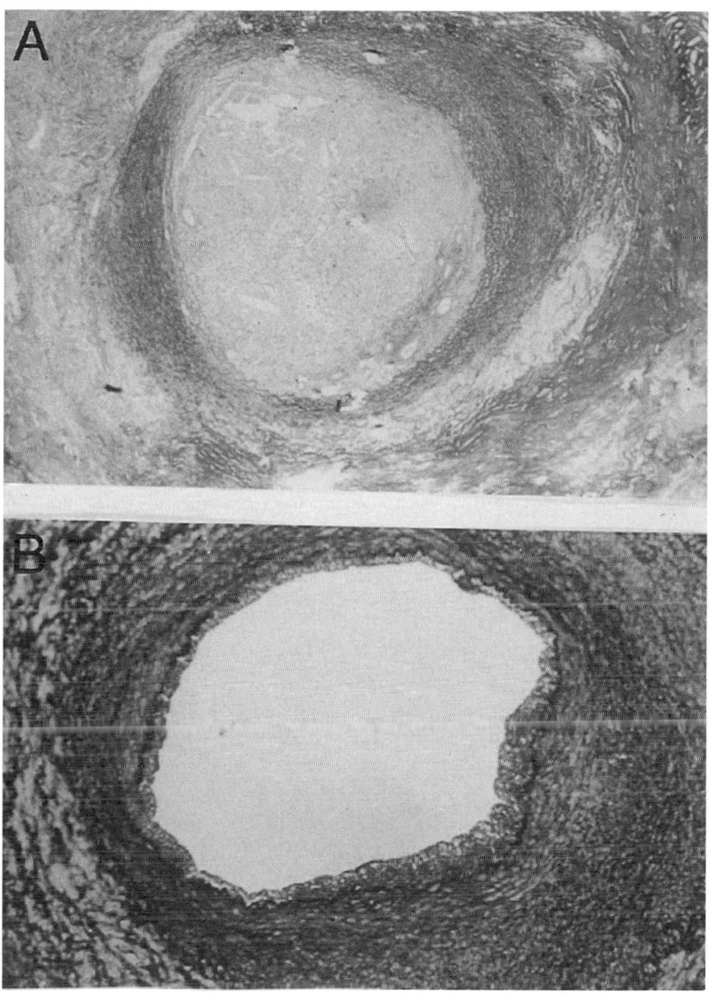

FIGURE 1.

Saphenous vein **(A)** and internal thoracic artery **(B)** grafts removed from the same patient undergoing heart transplantation four years after coronary surgery. The vein graft is occluded by a combination of intimal proliferation with superimposed thrombotic occlusion. The ITA lumen is well preserved, with minimal intimal proliferation above a clearly defined internal elastic lamina.

changes without significant morphologic change), to type II (endothelial denudation without intimal and medial damage), and, finally, to the most severe injury, type III (endothelial denudation with intimal and medial damage). Venous bypass grafts may be subject to type I and II injury and, potentially, focal areas of type III injury.[16]

Loss of endothelium eliminates the physical and electrostatic barrier separating platelets from subendothelial collagen, to which binding initiates platelet activation.[29] Loss of endothelial cells, or impairment of their function, leads to reduced production of prostacyclin,[30] nitric oxide,[31] and intrinsic fibrinolytic activity,[32] which act to inhibit platelet activation and adhesion and, hence, inhibit thrombus formation. Platelet activation stimulates synthesis of thromboxane A_2[33] and release of clear granule components, including platelet-derived growth factor (PDGF), platelet factor IV, fibrinogen, fibronectin, von Willebrand factor, and β-thromboglobulin.[34] These agents act together to produce vasoconstriction[35] and further platelet aggregation[33] and, hence, promote further generation of thrombin and fibrin. Early thrombotic occlusions within the first month after operation occur in 8% to 18% of saphenous vein grafts,[36] particularly under conditions of low flow, in the presence of an inadequate distal coronary circulation.

Within a few days of implantation, even when endothelial continuity is preserved, medial thickening occurs secondary to VSMC hyperplasia.[25, 37] These changes are the immediate response of the vessel wall to "injury" and are caused by release of growth factors, e.g., PDGF, fibroblast growth factor (FGF) from platelets, monocytes, and downregulation of the inhibitory effects of the intact endothelium. The realization that the behavior of the VSMC is central to this process has led to intense research toward achieving an understanding of the paracrine and autocrine influences that modulate its proliferative activity (Fig 2). Although many different stimuli interact to produce intimal hyperplasia, a range of growth factors are important in mediating proliferation of VSMCs.[15, 38] These growth factors are released from blood components, endothelial cells, and VSMCs themselves. After binding to cell surface receptors, they act to stimulate cell proliferation by signal transduction which leads to activation of intracellular second messenger systems, e.g., cyclic adenosine monophosphate (cAMP) and tyrosine kinase, which convert VSMCs from a quiescent to a proliferative phenotype.

Platelet-derived growth factor was originally shown to be released from platelets, but it is now known to be released from endothelial cells, VSMCs, fibroblasts, and macrophages.[38] Platelet-derived growth factor is chemotactic to monocytes and macrophages, but it is both chemotactic and mitogenic to VSMCs. It is undoubtedly important in the early response to injury, and infusion of recombinant PDGF BB has been shown to stimulate migration and proliferation of VSMCs in a rat model of angioplasty,[39] probably by separate pathways.[40] Recent data have also demonstrated that transfer of the PDGF BB isomer gene to the arterial wall results in intimal proliferation, thereby confirming the importance of PDGF as a stimulus to proliferation of VSMCs.[41] In a porcine model of vein grafts, increased expression of messenger RNA for PDGF B-chain, in association with the demonstration of a PDGF-like mitogen, was observed after endothelial regeneration, thereby supporting the role of PDGF in ongoing intimal hyperplasia.[42]

Fibroblast growth factors are a family of polypeptide molecules. The best-characterized molecules are the acidic (aFGF) and basic (bFGF) forms. Both forms are potent mitogens for a variety of cells, including endothelial cells and VSMCs.[38, 43] These cells are synthesized by endothelium, VSMCs, and monocytes; bound within the vessel wall to heparan sulfate to prevent degradation; and stored in the extracellular matrix.[44] After arterial wall injury, heparanases released from platelets and macrophages degrade the

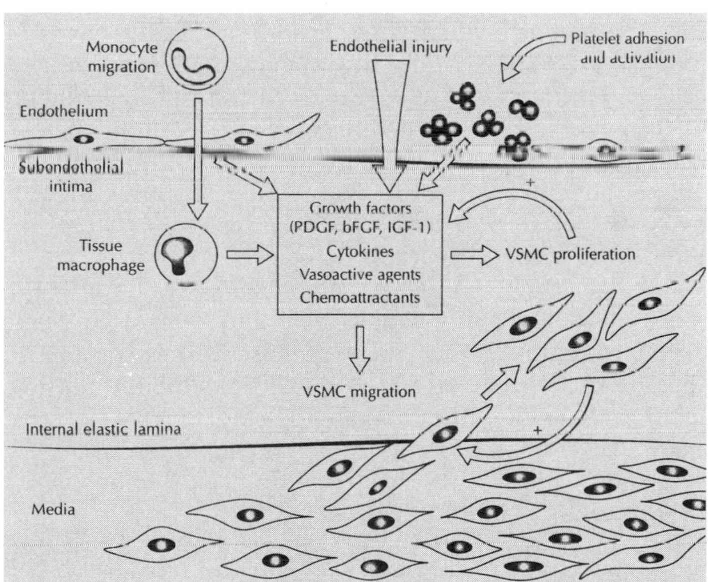

FIGURE 2.

Schematic representation of the cellular and biomolecular mediators involved in the acute response of the vessel wall to injury. *Abbreviations: PDGF,* platelet-derived growth factor; *bFGF,* basic fibroblast growth factor; *IGF-1,* insulin-like growth factor (Modified from Bryan AJ, Angelini GO: The biology of saphenous vein graft occlusion: Etiology and strategies for prevention. *Curr Opin Cardiol* 9:641–649, 1994.)

extracellular matrix, thereby releasing bFGF. In experimental models of arterial injury, exogenously administered bFGF caused proliferation of VSMCs in the presence of endothelial injury[45] and antibody to bFGF inhibited proliferation of VSMCs but did not reduce the overall degree of intimal thickening.[46] Further, recent data have shown that direct gene transfer of aFGF to the arterial wall produced intimal hyperplasia in a porcine model, thereby confirming its role in VSMC proliferation.[47] It also seems that bFGF has a role in re-establishing an endothelial lining in denuded vessels.[48] Currently, its importance in human vein graft disease remains to be established.

A number of other growth factors (insulin-like growth factor [IGF-1], transforming growth factor (TGF)-α and -β, and epidermal growth factor) and their receptors, which may be important in intimal hyperplasia, have been identified.[15, 38] Insulin-like growth factor is secreted by endothelial cells, VSMCs, and macrophages.[38] Receptors for IGF-1 binding have been demonstrated in human saphenous vein[49]; however, the importance of this in vein graft disease has not yet been elucidated. In additon, several vasoactive substances and cytokines, including angiotensin, endothelins, prostacyclin, and nitric oxide, appear to exert controlling influences over the proliferative and contractile status of VSMCs.[15] The cytokines, including interleukins and tumor necrosis factor, are emerging as an important mechanism of intercellular signaling among leucocytes, endothelial cells, and VSMCs and may play a part in the development of intimal hyperplasia in vein grafts.[15]

Vascular smooth muscle cells express a number of early-response genes (c-*fos*, c-*jun*, c-*myc*, and c-*myb*) in response to growth factor stimulation. The expression of these proto-oncogenes is thought to be involved in the signal transduction pathways that lead to cell proliferation. In angioplasty models, expression of c-*myc* and c-*fos* messenger RNA occurs early after injury.[50, 51] Early expression of these genes has recently been demonstrated in human saphenous vein after harvesting.[52]

The early response to injury is then followed for several weeks by a phase during which VSMCs undergo a change from a contractile to a proliferative phenotype[53] and then migrate from the media through the internal elastic lamina into the intima. A phase of rapid intimal proliferation then occurs.[26] Intimal hyperplasia is a chronic structural change that occurs in saphenous vein grafts. It is defined as the abnormal migration and proliferation of VSMCs with associated deposition of extracellular connective tissue matrix.[16] Subsequently, proliferation of VSMCs slows, and secretion and deposition of extracellular matrix accounts in part for the further increases in wall thickening.[26] The hypothesis that the degree of early proliferation of VSMCs is related to platelet deposition[54] is supported by its reduction in an animal model made thrombocytopenic.[55] Intimal proliferation continues well after endothelial regeneration and termination of platelet activation, however, which suggests that the autocrine and paracrine influences of the endothelium and VSMCs are important.[56]

Intimal proliferation continues for many months, and experimental work supports the view that the degree of late intimal hyperplasia is not influenced by the severity of the endothelial injury at the time of implantation.[26] By 1 year after implantation, the luminal diameter of saphenous vein grafts may have been reduced by 25%, primarily by intimal thickening.[19] After the first month, vein graft occlusion also results from thrombosis, but this is increasingly superimposed on a graft lumen narrowed by intimal proliferation. During this later phase, there are marked increases in the connective tissue matrix consequent on the secretory activity of the VSMCs and fibroblasts, with further thickening of both the media and intima.[26] Although the extracellular matrix provides both mechanical and structural support, component macromolecules, like the proteoglycans, interact with surrounding VSMCs to influence their differentiation, metabolism, migration, and proliferation.[57,58] Matrix degradation in response to injury relieves the inhibitory controls on VSMCs. The initial step in this process is the secretion of matrix metalloproteinases, which are enzymes of the endopeptidase family. In models of angioplasty[59] and vein grafts,[60] expression of metalloproteinases is upregulated. In saphenous vein grafts, secretion of extracellular matrix by synthetic VSMCs constitutes a major proportion of the wall thickening that occurs, particularly in the later phase. The important role of the matrix is increasingly being recognized, and modulation of the secretory activity of VSMCs is a further potential strategy to inhibit intimal hyperplasia.

Between the first and fourth years after implantation, limited changes may occur, with an occlusion rate of only 2% per year.[14] There is less cellular activity, and the lumen to wall thickness ratio stabilizes. There may be an increase in the lipid content and the number of foam cells that may be precursors of atherosclerosis. Perhaps most importantly, intimal hyperplasia may be seen as a predisposing factor and a precursor of atheroma formation. It is reasonable to speculate that the location of atheroma in vein grafts is determined by similar factors and occurs preferentially at sites of intimal thickening. In both human beings and animal models, intimal hyperplasia precedes atheroma formation in vein grafts,[61] and fatty infiltration stimulates further proliferation of VSMCs, thereby eventually resulting in atheroma formation.[38]

Atherosclerotic changes are seen at 3 years and accelerate beyond 5 years with the appearance of mature lipid-laden atherosclerotic plaques, when the rate of graft occlusion is approximately 5% per year.[14] The appearance of the atherosclerotic process in vein grafts is very similar to that seen in arteries. Overall, it may be more friable and diffuse, but it is rarely calcified and may result in aneurysmal dilatation, plaque rupture, and superimposed thrombus leading to sudden graft occlusion and clinical ischemic events.[19] By 10 years, approximately 50% of grafts are occluded, and most others have evidence of significant vein graft disease.[14] This finding contrasts markedly with the situation in ITA grafts: After an early occlusion rate of 5% to 10%, the remaining grafts are patent at 10 years with no evidence of progressive degeneration.[6]

FACTORS INFLUENCING GRAFT PATENCY

Many factors influence graft patency; the biological characteristics of the conduit used, the technical aspects of the surgical procedure, and the anatomy and disease of the coronary circulation are factors of primary importance. No matter how favorable the biological characteristics of a conduit may be, however, the techical aspects of the surgical procedure must always be considered to formulate its appropriate place in clinical practice.

BIOLOGICAL CHARACTERISTICS OF CONDUITS

The relevant biological characteristics of conduits used for coronary bypass are (1) the antithrombotic properties of the conduit and, in particular, the behavior of the vascular endothelium; (2) the tendency of the conduit to have intimal thickening and late atherosclerotic change develop when implanted into the coronary circulation; and (3) the ability of the chosen conduit to respond to the changing requirements of the coronary circulation.[62] These differences are greatest between arteries and veins; nevertheless, there are major differences among autologous arteries in their ability to resist atherosclerotic change and respond to vasoactive stimuli in the same individual, despite exposure to the same atherogenic stimuli and circulating agents.[63]

Saphenous Vein Grafts

Intrinsic Properties.—It is becoming increasingly clear, mainly from clinical investigations in the peripheral vascular field, that the intrinsic qualities of the saphenous vein may have an important bearing on its successful use in arterial reconstruction.[64, 65] Veins with reduced compliance,[64] pre-existing intimal hyperplasia, or other histologic abnormalities[65] are at increased risk of early graft stenoses and failure. In particular, the presence of subendothelial spindle-shaped cells greater than five layers thick appears to be associated with a poor outcome.[66] In addition, VSMCs from patients who have stenoses caused by intimal hyperplasia appear to exhibit decreased sensitivity to heparin inhibition when cultured in vitro, which suggests differences in the proliferative behavior of VSMCs from different individuals.[67, 68] Angioscopic identification of an increased number of intraluminal abnormalities in cephalic vein has provided an explanation for the previously poor outcome associated with the use of upper limb veins for arterial reconstruction.[69]

Response to Injury.—The pathophysiologic changes that may occur during the mobilization, preparation, and storage of long saphenous vein before its implantation have been well described.[70, 71] Endothelial loss and impairment of the metabolic integrity of the media may be demonstrated both morphologically and functionally.[72–76] There are a number of different mechanisms of injury: mechanical, resulting directly from the surgical manipulation; ischemic, caused by interruption of *vasa vasorum*; temperature; chemical, resulting from the storage solution; pressure, resulting from excessive intraluminal distension.[70] Of these, excessive distension has been shown to be detrimental to early graft patency in an animal model.[25] Recent work has furthered our understanding of the effect of surgical preparation on saphenous vein. The intrinsic fibrinolytic activity of the saphenous vein is impaired by surgical preparation potentially favoring thrombosis.[32] Early intimal proliferation is enhanced after surgical preparation in organ culture, which suggests an increased sensitivity to mitogenic stimuli.[77, 78] In addition, after preparation, the vasoreactivity of saphenous vein grafts to a variety of vasoconstrictors is diminished in absolute terms, although with apparently increased relative sensitivity.[79]

The basic message remains unchanged: Damage to the vein at the time of surgical preparation has a number of detrimental effects that favor early thrombotic occlusion, although these effects do not appear to influence the degree of late intimal hyperplasia.

Response to Hemodynamic Factors.—Vein grafts interposed into the arterial circulation experience a profound change in the hemodynamic forces to which they are exposed. It is generally accepted that this change stimulates proliferation of VSMCs and that some degree of intimal thickening and wall thickening is an adaptive response to these forces. Among these forces, wall tension appears to be of paramount importance,[80–82] although discussion in relation to the importance of other variables, such as shear stress, continues.[83] The mechanisms by which hemodynamic change results in biological response are currently being elucidated. The vascular endothelial cell can respond to stretching forces, which are probably transduced by a stretch-activated channel on the endothelial-cell surface.[84] These stresses then activate second messenger systems, inducing endothelial-cell gene transcription of PDGF[85, 86] and, potentially, other paracrine mitogenic substances, which transform hemodynamic stimulus into adaptive vascular wall response. In addition to the proliferative response, hemodynamic stresses also lead to increased synthesis of collagen, elastin, and matrix components.[87, 88] It might therefore be anticipated that methods aimed at reducing wall tension represent a potentially effective strategy to inhibit intimal hyperplasia.

Autologous Arterial Conduits

Intrinsic Properties.—It comes as no great surprise that autologous arteries function better as arterial replacements than does reversed saphenous vein. In general, most such comparisons are between the ITA and other conduits because of its superior performance and frequent use. The ITA produces prostacyclin and nitric oxide in greater amounts than does saphenous vein.[89, 90] Indeed, other autologous conduits also release these substances in greater quantities than does saphenous vein, including the gastroepiploic and inferior epigastric arteries.[91] There is also some evidence to suggest that the differences in graft patency may even be determined by selection of different regions of an arterial graft. The distal ITA not only has a smaller caliber, it also exhibits markedly greater contractility,[92] which indicates that there may be a biological explanation for the reduced patency of grafts involving the ITA bifurcation.[93] These characteristics therefore provide a powerful mechanism to protect against spasm and inhibit platelet aggregation and VSMC proliferation.

Intimal thickening does not develop in ITA grafts to any significant degree. The response of VSMCs from saphenous vein exhibits a marked proliferative response to pulsatile stretch compared with VSMCs from the ITA in isolated cell culture.[94] In addition, PDGF stimulates proliferation of venous VSMCs to a much greater degree than those obtained from the ITA.[62, 63] Similarly, surgical preparation appears to act as a definite stimulus to VSMC proliferation in saphenous vein in organ culture compared with the ITA, which suggests differences in the behavior of these two conduits in response to injury.[95] The differences in the response to mitogenic stimuli may at least be explained in part by the observation in a canine model of increased high-affinity receptor sites for bFGF in saphenous vein compared with ITA, a difference that is further increased by subjecting the venous tissue to excessive intraluminal distension.[96]

The susceptibility of different autologous arteries to atherosclerotic change also varies. A clear understanding of the biological properties can therefore be used not only to explain the differences in clinical behavior but also to predict the performance of some of the more recently introduced arterial conduits.[97, 98] It has been suggested that the multiple elastic lamellae and absence of discontinuities in the internal elastic lamina of the ITA provide relative protection against intimal thickening and atherosclerotic change.[97, 99] The observation that the gastroepiploic, inferior epigastric, and radial arteries have fewer elastic lamellae and more discontinuities has led some investigators to predict a greater tendency to intimal hyperplasia and a potentially worse long-term outcome with these conduits in comparison with the ITA.[97, 99]

Flow Patterns and Responses.—The pattern of flow through arterial grafts is substantially different from that through vein grafts. Although vein grafts exhibit predominantly diastolic flow patterns throughout their length, pedicled arterial grafts show a transition from a predominantly systolic pattern proximally to a more marked diastolic component distally.[100] Not only is the rise in the diastolic flow velocity more sustained, but the absolute flow velocity is also greater in ITA grafts compared with saphenous vein grafts,[100] with resultant secondary differences in wall tension and shear stress. Absolute flow through ITA grafts is also substantially lower than that through vein grafts,[101] and hypoperfusion syndromes are well recognized either in association with spasm[102, 103] or, particularly, when diseased vein grafts are replaced with arterial grafts at reoperation.[104]

Flow-dependent vasodilation is observed in ITA grafts but not in saphenous vein grafts under high output conditions, such as atrial pacing.[105] Shear stress changes at the blood-endothelial interface may stimulate production of nitric oxide, which mediates this phenomenon and contributes to the ability of arterial bypass grafts to respond to increased myocardial blood flow requirements.[62, 63] It also seems that these beneficial aspects of endothelial function persist when arterial conduits are used as free grafts.[106]

Among the available arterial conduits, there is a variation in response of the ITA, gastroepiploic artery, and inferior epigastric artery (IEA) to a range of vasoconstrictors, which are either endogenous mediators of vascular tone or drugs administered during cardiac surgical procedures.[107] These differences represent a combination of the receptor profiles and the muscle and elastin content of the range of available conduits. This finding has led He and associates[100] to propose a functional classification of arterial grafts: type I (somatic arteries), type II (splanchnic arteries), and type III (limb arteries). Types II and III include the radial and gastroepiploic arteries and are prone to spasm, whereas type I arteries, like the ITA and IEA, are usually less prone to spasm. It therefore seems that there are clear differences in flow regarding pattern, magnitude, and the flow responses in different physiologic situations between the range of arterial and venous conduits. The precise relation between these observed differences and long-term clinical performance is not clearly defined.

THE CORONARY CIRCULATION

Physiologic and anatomical aspects of the coronary circulation significantly influence graft patency. When the patency rates for grafts to the three principal coronary territories—LAD, right, and circumflex—are analyzed, clear differences emerge. Grafts to the LAD coronary artery have the highest patency rates, regardless of the conduit used.[108, 109] In fact, equivalent early patency rates for saphenous vein and ITA grafts to the LAD have been demonstrated when factors, including vessel size, graft flow, and degree of native vessel stenosis, were controlled for.[110] In several studies, grafts to the circumflex and right coronary systems have emerged as independent predictors of reduced early patency.[109, 111] Although one potential reason for such a finding may be the differences in flow within the different vessels, it is also impossible to refute the argument that constructing grafts to the inferior and posterior surfaces of the heart is simply more difficult and therefore more susceptible to technical error.[109]

The size of the grafted artery has also been identified as a risk factor for early occlusion. Target arteries with an intraluminal diameter of less than 1.5 mm, diffuse disease, or distal vessels poorly visible or invisible at angiography are at increased risk of early occlusion.[109, 111, 112] These characteristics, in an indirect way, emphasise the importance of adequate flow in maintaining graft patency.

TECHNICAL SURGICAL CONSIDERATIONS

Although the above factors are important, it must be acknowledged that individual surgical skill is an important determinant of graft patency. Indeed, a significant difference in operative mortality has been observed among individual surgeons, which may not be explained by patient-related variables.[113] The best results are achieved by those surgeons and institutions performing coronary artery in sufficient volume to develop and maintain their expertise.[113, 114] Although this has always been a sensitive area to discuss and investigate, Bex et al.[115] have elegantly demonstrated that such factors cannot be ignored, however complex the statistical analysis.

Surgical factors are also of greater importance when the more complex and demanding procedures, which require multiple arterial conduits, are involved. Major differences in graft patency have been observed between groups with a small experience[116] and those with a large experience[117] in the use of the inferior epigastric artery graft. The message here is simple yet important. Whatever the biological characteristics of a graft, if the factors associated with its mobilization or implantation are technically challenging, then patency and clinical outcome may suffer. Only the individual surgeon can judge the operative strategy that is likely to yield the best early and late outcome given the prevailing circumstances.

SYSTEMIC INFLUENCES

A number of systemic influences affect late graft atherosclerosis and patency. These influences predominantly affect vein grafts, thus illustrating a further difference, namely, the susceptibility of the range of conduits to extrinsic influences. Implantation of vein grafts into the arterial circulation leads to lipid accumulation in the vessel wall in primates,[118] but whether this effect in itself represents a stimulus to intimal proliferation is still controversial. In a rabbit model, hypercholesterolemia enhanced intimal hyperplasia,[119] but increased cholesterol accumulation in primate vein grafts did not enhance intimal thickening.[118] Patients who have disordered lipid-cholesterol metabolism and are undergoing coronary bypass grafting are at increased risk of vein graft atherosclerosis and occlusion, which leads to further intervention.[120] In patients who have atherosclerotic grafts, total serum levels of cholesterol and triglycerides are higher than in those who have vein grafts that are apparently free of disease.[120] In addition, the level of high density lipoprotein cholesterol is lower and the level of low density lipoprotein cholesterol is higher in patients who have atherosclerotic grafts.[120] A further clinical study has demonstrated an association between serum levels of lipoprotein A and an increased risk of saphenous vein graft stenosis.[121] It is also possible that the association between hypercoagulability and high levels of triglyceride levels may be implicated in the late risk of graft thrombosis.[122] These data suggest that the relationship between disordered lipid profile and late graft failure is strong, even in comparison to other atherogenic factors, like smoking.[123] Neither total serum levels of cholesterol nor levels of triglyceride, however, have been found to be predictive of long-term survival in patients undergoing coronary artery surgery.[124] Smoking is clearly associated with increased cardiovascular morbidity and mortality, and higher graft occlusion rates have been documented in smokers.[125] The exact mechanisms remain uncertain, and a discussion of these is outside the scope of this text.

STRATEGIES TO IMPROVE GRAFT PATENCY

The observation that graft failure is a multifactorial process that may develop over a prolonged period leads to the conclusion that a rational approach to optimizing graft patency is likely to incorporate a number of components.

ARTERIAL GRAFTS

Surgical Preparation

The question of injury to arterial grafts during preparation has generally received far less attention compared with vein grafts, presumably because surgeons perceive this to be less of a problem, given the excellent early results achieved with left ITA grafting. Endothelial injury is rarely seen in arterial grafts during preparation,[126] although injudicious use of electrocautery may result in endothelial injury and mural thrombus formation.[127] Preparation techniques that demand intraluminal instrumentation, either for dilatation or administration of vasodilating agents, are best avoided, because any beneficial effects are uncertain and there must be a risk of endothelial-intimal injury.[128] Distension of the ITA has been shown to reduce production of prostacyclin in an animal model.[129] Far more catastrophic than these types of injury is localized or generalized dissection, which has been reported both locally[130] and generally in the ITA and may even result in early postoperative death.[131] With careful preparation and accurate implantation, therefore, the favorable biological characteristics of arterial grafts protect against early thrombotic occlusion.

Antithrombotic Agents

Studies of the influence of antithrombotic agents, particularly antiplatelet agents such as aspirin, have not been shown to have any significant influence on early ITA graft patency.[132] There is very limited information on the influence of these agents on the performance of alternative arterial conduits. It is perhaps not surprising to find that the superior intrinsic antithrombotic properties of arterial conduits, coupled with a low risk of early thrombotic occlusion via platelet-mediated mechanisms, mean that antiplatelet agents do not produce any demonstrable therapeutic effect.

VEIN GRAFTS

Early Failure

Surgical Factors.—Efforts to improve early graft patency have centereed on the use of surgical techniques during harvesting and implantation that maintain the structural and functional integrity of the saphenous vein.[133–135] Surgical injury can be prevented by minimizing mechanical trauma and avoiding overdistension. Several methods have been proposed to achieve this goal. The use of a cocktail of long-acting vasodilators is reported to result in excellent vasodilatation without the use of hydrostatic force.[136] Simple modifications to the bypass circuit may also limit the distension of the vein to physiologic pressures and in so doing allow preparation of vein grafts with intact structure and function.[137, 138]

The influence of surgical damage on early graft patency in human coronary bypass grafting has not been clearly defined. Data from animal models have indicated that overdistension may lead to a reduction in early graft patency[25] but has little influence on the later degree of intimal hyperplasia.[26] Nevertheless, clinical trials are unlikely to be considered ethical, and the observations that the detrimental effects observed during preparation of the saphenous vein all appear to favor thrombotic occlusion suggest that every effort should be reasonably made to eliminate these influences at the time of surgery.

Antithrombotic Agents.—The use of antithrombotic agents to reduce the risk of early thrombotic occlusion of vein grafts has been accepted practice since the trials reported in the early 1980s.[139] In the interim period, the place of antiplatelet agents in maintaining graft patency has been clarified, and several useful meta-analyses have been presented.[140–142] On the basis of available evidence, 100–325 mg aspirin per day started in the early postoperative period represents the lowest dose with a consistent antithrombotic effect.[140, 141] There is little evidence that additional antiplatelet agents, such as dipyridamole, result in further improvements in graft patency, although other antiplatelet agents have been shown to be as effective as aspirin.[141, 143] Oral anticoagulant therapy, such as warfarin (coumadin), appears to be as effective but not more so.[141, 142, 144] The use of oral anticoagulants in special situations, i.e., after endarterectomy, is not supported by the available data, which although limited appear to favor aspirin.[145, 146] The use of aspirin in conjunction with anticoagulants and the possible additive benefits are ill defined, and further work in this area may be of value. Data from the Veterans Affairs Cooperative Study indicated that, overall, aspirin did not affect graft patency 1–3 years after operation, presumalby because it fails to suppress proliferation of VSMCs.[147] Nevertheless, aspirin should be continued indefinitely, given its proven role as secondary prevention against cardiovascular events.[148,149]

Late Failure

Pharmacologic Approaches.—A variety of pharmacologic agents have been evaluated in a range of animal models; these models have been reviewed in detail elsewhere.[15–17] To summarize, there is currently no effective pharmacologic therapy to prevent vein graft disease. Heparin and low–molecular weight (LMW) heparin, despite theoretical potential and a demonstrable effect on VSMC in vitro,[150] have been disappointing in both organ culture and animal models of vein grafts.[151, 152] Clinical trials in angioplasty restenosis have yielded negative results,[153] although a trial of patients undergoing coronary bypass has not been conducted. A trial of LMW heparin in patients undergoing peripheral vascular reconstruction showed improved graft patency in the LMW heparin group.[154] No assessment of intimal hyperplasia was made, and these effects could be attributed to anticoagulant rather than antiproliferative effects. Calcium channel blockers, angiopeptin, and angiotensin-converting enzyme (ACE) inhibitors have all been shown to retard intimal hyperplasia in animal models of vein grafts.[14–16] Preliminary reports of a reduction in vein graft disease but not patency in a clinical trial of calcium antagonists after coronary surgery[155] remain unconfirmed, although the demonstration that these agents inhibit proliferation of VSMCs caused by PDGF but not by wall tension suggests that their potential in this area is limited.[156] In the clinical arena, ACE inhibitors and angiopeptin have both been ineffective in improving outcome after angioplasty.[157, 158] There have been no reports of their clinical evaluation in patients after coronary surgery. Newer agents that inhibit the Na^+-H^+ exchanger, a membrane transport protein activated by growth factors as an early event when VSMCs enter the cell cycle, appear effective in animal models of arterial injury[159, 160] but have not been evaluated in vein grafts.

Lipid lowering therapy is the only pharmacologic approach with at least some proven benefit in a clinical setting. The combination of colestipol and niacin has been shown to reduce the incidence of new lesion formation but not graft patency in patients who have had previous coronary artery bypass grafts.[161, 162] The effects demonstrated can at best be considered modest, and National Institutes of Heath trials are currently under way to evaluate the role of hepatic hydroxymethylglutaryl coenzyme A reductase inhibitors and aspirin in combination with lipid lowering therapy in the prevention of vein graft atherosclerosis.[123]

External Vessel Supports.—This strategy is based on the observed importance of wall tension in stimulating proliferation of VSMCs after implantation of vein grafts. The hypothesis, therefore, is that an external vessel support created by reducing wall tension may reduce adaptive wall thickening. Several studies with different stents in a number of animal models have shown a reduction in intimal thickening.[163, 164] Our own initial investigations, however, with a restrictive polytetrafluoroethylene stent indicated that although medial proliferation was reduced, intimal proliferation and luminal encroachment were greater in the stented grafts.[165] More recent investigations in an established porcine model have shown marked reductions in medial and intimal thickening in grafts stented extravascularly with initially nonrestrictive 6 or 8 mm porous Dacron grafts with external helical polythene supports (Fig 3).[166] The improvements in luminal cross-sectional area and reductions in medial and intimal cross-sectional area persisted regardless of stent size,[167] and there was reduced cellular proliferative activity in the vessel wall of stented grafts.[166] The porous nature of this stent should have minimal effects on fluid flux and permit unhindered growth of a neoadventitia. The size of the stent was chosen to allow unrestricted expansion of the graft in initial response to arterial pressure. Subsequent incorporation of the stent in the neoadventitia might then reduce tangential wall stress and consequently reduce medial thickening and intima formation. The results of long-term animal implants are awaited, but the data would indicate that a clinical trial should be conducted to evaluate this approach completely.

Photodynamic Therapy.—This technique uses the ability of light excitable photosensitizers to produce injury to targeted cells, in this case VSMCs, when activated by the appropriate wavelength of light. Photodynamic therapy has been shown to be an effective inhibitor of intimal hyperplasia in an animal model of arterial injury[168] and in an in vitro culture system of VSMCs.[169] Recent

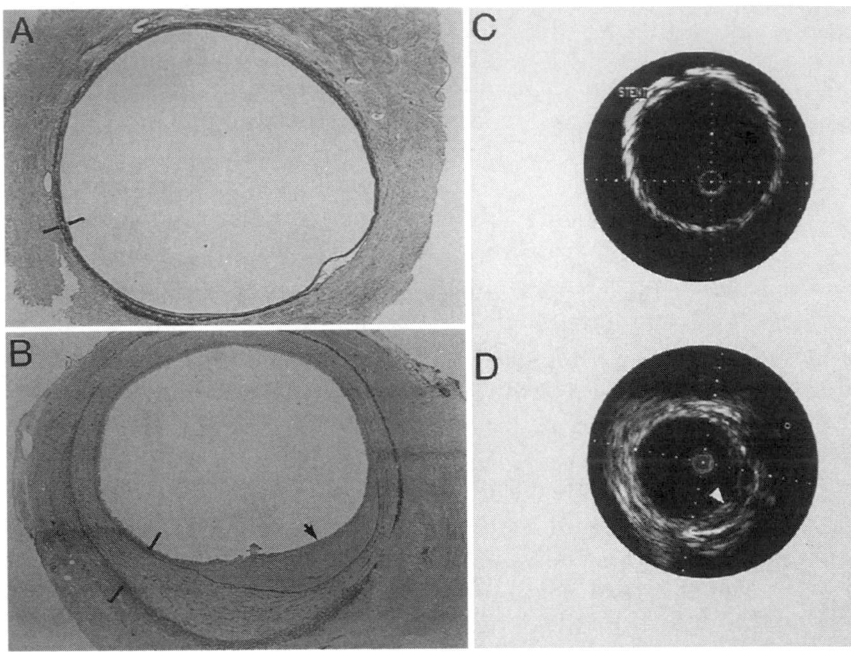

FIGURE 3.

Transverse sections of experimental vein grafts with an extravascular stent **(A)** and without a stent **(B).** There is a significantly greater degree of intimal hyperplasia *(arrow)* and wall thickness *(between bars)* in unstented porcine grafts. Companion intravascular ultrasound images of stented **(C)** and unstented **(D)** grafts with prominent intimal hyperplasia *(arrow)* in the unstented graft.

data in a model of rat jugular vein to carotid artery grafting have demonstrated for the first time a reduction in intimal hyperplasia in the body of these grafts; unfortunately, the degree of intimal thickening that occurred at the anastomotic sites was unchanged.[170] Further information on this interesting approach should be forthcoming, although whether the cumbersome nature of these light exposure techniques prevents their practical clinical application remains to be seen.

Molecular Biological Approaches.—The rapid developments in molecular biology have opened the way to a whole new range of potential strategies for the inhibition of intimal hyperplasia.[15, 17, 18] Much of the work in this area has focused on responses to arterial injury, with particular reference to restenosis after angioplasty. Nevertheless, the potential use of these techniques with vein grafts offers the unique opportunity for topical therapy at the time of implantation. These techniques might be used to modify the biological behavior of conduits so that they resist factors promoting both early and late occlusion. For the sake of clarity, these techniques are presented together in this section. Several different approaches are possible (Figs 4 and 5).[15, 17, 18]

Antibody-Specific Inhibition.—Specific antibodies raised to growth factors have been applied in models of arterial injury directed against both PDGF and b-FGF (Fig 4). A polyclonal anti-PDGF IgG reduced intimal hyperplasia after balloon injury in the rat carotid injury model; its mechanism of action appeared predominantly to be by prevention of migration rather than proliferation.[171] Similarly, antibodies to bFGF reduced proliferation of VSMCs but not the overall degree of intimal hyperplasia in the rat angioplasty model.[172] The main defects in any strategy directed against a specific growth factor are the multiple paracrine influences on intimal hyperplasia; thus, only partial suppression can ever result from inhibition of a single growth factor.

A different approach has been to target the extracellular matrix. Cell binding to matrix is mediated by cell surface receptors

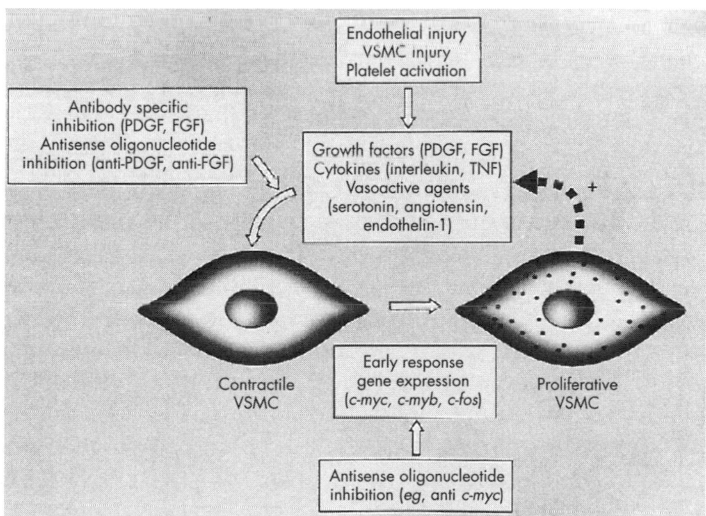

FIGURE 4.

Potential molecular biological strategies for inhibiting intimal hyperplasia. (Modified from Bryan AJ, Angelini GD: The biology of saphenous vein graft occlusion: Etiology and strategies for prevention. *Curr Opin Cardiol* 9:641–649, 1994.)

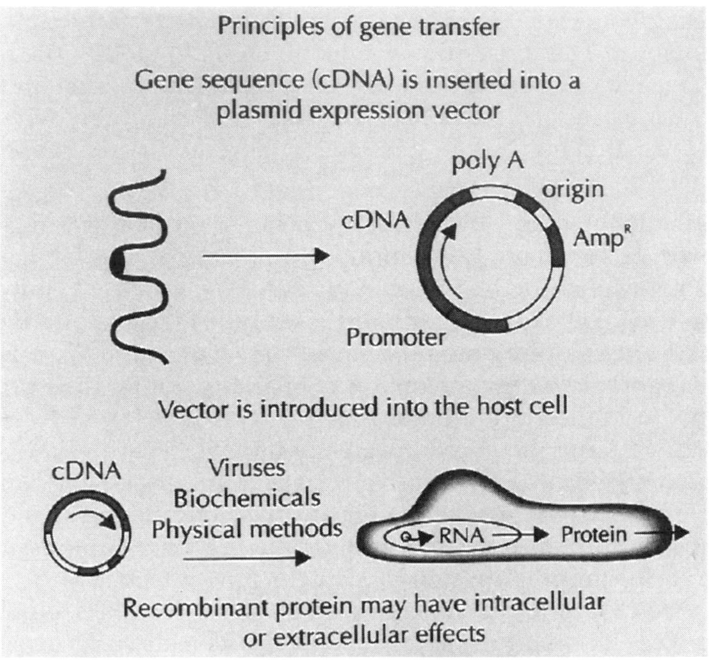

FIGURE 5.

Principles of gene transfer. *Abbreviations: AmpR,* ampicillin resistance; *cDNA,* complementary DNA; *Poly A,* noncoding repetitive sequence of adenine. (Adapted from Nabel EG, Pomplili VJ, Plantz GE, et al: Gene transfer and vascular disease. *Cardiovasc Res* 28:445–455, 1994.)

called integrins. A monoclonal antibody to an integrin($a_v b_3$) and an integrin receptor antagonist have been used to inhibit migration of VSMCs in vitro.[173]

New approaches to the use of antithrombotic agents are also being developed. One approach has been to target fibrinolytic therapy to the vessel wall.[174] Preliminary data have been presented to show a reduction of thrombus formation in an experimental model in which LMW urokinase was linked to a monoclonal antibody bound to damaged endothelium.[175] Locally bound thrombolytic agents could provide intense but localized anticoagulation and might be useful in maintaining graft patency. Further developments of this kind of approach are awaited with interest.

Antisense Oligonucleotide Inhibition.—This approach involves the development of antisense oligonucleotides with complementary base sequences that bind to a specific messenger RNA and, in so doing, inhibit its translation (Fig 4).[18] In cultures of VSMCs and endothelial cells, antisense oligonucleotides to messenger RNA for PDGF-A, bFGF, and transforming growth factor-β, introduced with the use of liposome-mediated transfection, appeared to block production of these factors effectively.[176] Antisense oligonucleotides to both *c-myc* and *c-myb* proto-oncogenes have been shown to inhibit proliferation of VSMCs both in vitro and in vivo in models of arterial injury.[177, 178] Other proteins implicated in proliferation of VSMCs, such as proliferating cell nuclear antigen and nonmuscle myosin heavy chain, have also been inhibited by antisense technology.[179] The recent demonstration that expression of *c-fos* and *c-myc* is triggered by harvesting saphenous vein[52] and successful inhibition of proliferation of VSMCs from human saphenous vein in vitro[180] means that this attractive approach requires further evaluation.

It would be wrong not to at least mention some of the difficulties.[18] For example, oligonucleotides enter cells by simple diffusion and are not targeted to specific cell types. High local concentrations and prolonged contact time may be required to achieve a meaningful biological response. Oligonucleotides have a relatively short half-life, and their ability to produce prolonged gene expression needs to be elucidated further. Finally, an improved understanding of both the action of oligonucleotides on vascular cells and the ability to differentiate nonspecific inhibitory effects on cells is required.

Gene Therapy.—This rapidly developing area may potentially be used to treat a range of vascular diseases.[18] Several different approaches can be used to correct the function of a defective gene or augment gene expression. In the United States, gene augmentation is used in most human disease protocols. This approach entails the introduction of a copy of the new gene into the host genome; the genes within the host cells are left intact. The two main approaches are direct gene transfer and cell-mediated gene transfer. With direct gene transfer, genes are directly transferred into the cells of the vessel wall (Fig 5). Genes can be transferred into cells by a number of different vectors, e.g., viruses and liposomes. In a range of animal models, gene transfer to the arterial wall has been accomplished with demonstrable expression up to 5 months.[18] At present, refinement of the technique is required to improve the efficiency of gene transfer and expression and to target genes to specific cells.[18] Cell-mediated gene transfer involves the in vitro modification of a cell line with subsequent in vivo implantation. Autologous endothelial cells have been modified in vitro with the use of recombinant retroviruses; evidence of effective repopulation by modified endothelial cells was observed 1–14 days after arterial injury in an animal model.[181] Effective viral transfer of vascular cell adhesion molecules, which may inhibit intimal hyperplasia by blocking endothelial monocyte adhesion, has been demonstrated in carotid artery vein grafts in an animal model with a high level of in vivo expression at 3 days.[182] Although these techniques are still in their infancy, they hold great promise for the future.

CONCLUSIONS

The problems of vein graft failure and the superior clinical performance of arterial conduits are widely recognized. Only with a greater understanding of the biological changes that occur within the vessel wall has it been possible to elucidate the complex pathophysiology of graft failure. Similarly, biological differences among the alternative conduits for coronary surgery have provided a clear explanation for the observed differences in patency and have been used to predict the long-term clinical behavior of the more recently introduced arterial conduits. Despite increased understanding of VSMC biology, strategies to improve late vein graft failure have proved elusive. Future work in this area is likely to rely heavily on molecular biological techniques, not only to elucidate further the cellular and autocrine influences on intimal hyperplasia but also to develop specific therapeutic agents. With the development of these techniques, the practical goal of effective gene therapy for a range of cardiovascular diseases may be realized.

REFERENCES

1. Marwick C: Coronary bypass grafting: Economics, including rehabilitation. *Curr Opin Cardiol* 9:635–640, 1994.
2. United Kingdom Cardiac Surgical Register: Society of Cardiothoracic Surgeons of Great Britain and Ireland, 1993.
3. Weintraub WS, Jones EL, Craver JM, et al: Frequency of repeat coronary bypass or coronary angioplasty after coronary artery bypass surgery using saphenous venous grafts. *Am J Cardiol* 73:103–112, 1994.
4. Akins CW, Buckley MJ, Daggett WM, et al: Reoperative coronary grafting: Changing patient profiles, operative indications, techniques and results. *Ann Thorac Surg* 58:359–365, 1994.
5. Lytle B: Arterial grafts and reoperative coronary bypass surgery, in Angelini GD, Bryan AJ, Dion R (eds): *Arterial Conduits in Myocardial Revascularisation.* London, Edward Arnold, 1995, pp 170–181.
6. Loop FD, Lytle BW, Cosgrove DM, et al: Influence of the internal mammary artery graft on 10 year survival and other cardiac events. *N Engl J Med* 314:1–6, 1986.
7. Grover FL, Johnson RR, Marshall G, et al: Impact of mammary grafts

on coronary bypass operative mortality and morbidity. *Ann Thorac Surg* 57:559–569, 1994.

8. Edwards FH, Clark RE, Schwartz M: Impact of internal mammary artery conduits on operative mortality in coronary revascularization. *Ann Thorac Surg* 57:27–32, 1994.
9. Kirklin JW, et al: ACC/ACH guidelines and indications for the coronary artery bypass graft surgery. *Circulation* 83:1125–1173, 1991.
10. Loop FD, Lytle BW, Cosgrove DM: New arteries for old. *Circulation* 79:I-40s–I-45s, 1989.
11. Barner HB: New arterial conduits for coronary bypass surgery. *Semin Thorac Cardiovasc Surg* 6:76–80, 1994.
12. Dion R, Etienne PY, Verhelst R, et al: Bilateral mammary grafting; Clinical, functional and angiographic assessment in 400 consecutive patients. *Eur J Cardiothorac Surg* 7:287–294, 1993.
13. Izzat MB, West RR, Bryan AJ, et al: Coronary artery bypass surgery: Current practice in the United Kingdom. *Br Heart J* 71:382–385, 1994.
14. Campeau L, Enjalbert M, Lesperance J, et al: Atherosclerois and late clousre of aortocoronary saphenous vein grafts: Sequential angiographic studies at 2 weeks, 1 year, 5 to 7 years and 10 to 12 years after surgery. *Circulation* 68:II-1s–II-7s, 1983.
15. Foegh ML, Virmani R: Molecular biology of intimal proliferation, in Yacoub M, Popper J (eds): *Annual of Cardiac Surgery.* London, Current Science, 1994, pp 53–65.
16. Davies MG, Hagen P-O: Pathobiology of intimal hyperplasia. *Br J Surg* 81:1254–1269, 1994.
17. Bryan AJ, Angelini GD: The biology of saphenous vein graft occlusion: Etiology and strategies for prevention. *Curr Opin Cardiol* 9:641–649, 1994.
18. Nabel EG, Pompili VJ, Plautz GE, et al: Gene transfer and vascular disease. *Cardiovasc Res* 28:445–455, 1994.
19. Grondin CM, Thornton JC: The natural history of saphenous vein grafts, in Luscher T, Turina M, Braunwald E (eds): *Coronary Artery Graft Disease: Mechanisms and Prevention.* Berlin, Springer Verlag, 1994, pp 3–16.
20. Bulkley BH, Hutchins GM: Accelerated atherosclerosis: A morphological study in 97 saphenous vein grafts. *Circulation* 55:163–169, 1977.
21. Bulkley BH, Hutchins GM: Pathology of coronary artery bypass graft surgery. *Arch Pathol Lab Med* 102:273–280, 1978.
22. Kalan JM, Roberts WC: Morphologic findings in saphenous veins used as coronary arterial bypass conduits for longer than one year: Necropsy analysis of 53 patients, 123 saphenous veins, and 1865 five-millimeter segments of veins. *Am Heart J* 119:1164–1184, 1990.
23. Cox JL, Chiasson DA, Gotlieb AI: Stranger in a strange land: The pathogenesis of saphenous vein graft stenosis with emphasis on structural and functional differences between veins and arteries. *Prog Cardiovasc Dis* 34:45–68, 1991.
24. Boerboom LE, Olinger GN, Lui T-Z, et al: Histologic, morphometric

and biochemical evaluation of vein bypass grafts in a non-human primate model: I. Sequential changes within the first three months. *J Thorac Cardiovasc Surg* 99:97–106, 1990.

25. Angelini GD, Bryan AJ, Williams HMJ, et al: Distention promotes platelet and leucocyte adhesion and reduces short term patency in pig arteriovenous bypass grafts. *J Thorac Cardiovasc Surg* 99:433–439, 1990.
26. Angelini GD, Bryan AJ, Williams HMJ, et al: Time course of medial and intimal thickening in pig venous arterial grafts: Relationship to endothelial injury and cholesterol accumulation. *J Thorac Cardiovasc Surg* 103:1093–1103, 1992.
27. Ip JH, Fuster V, Badimon L, et al: Syndromes of accelerated atherosclerosis: Role of vascular injury and smooth muscle cell proliferation. *J Am Coll Cardiol* 15:1667–1687, 1990.
28. Ross R: The pathogenesis of atherosclerosis: an update. *N Engl J Med* 314:488–500, 1986.
29. Baumgartner HR, Muggli R, Tschopp RB, et al: Platelet adhesion, release and aggregation in flowing blood: Effect of surface properties and platelet function. *Thromb Haemostas* 35:124–138, 1976.
30. Angelini GD, Breckenridge IM, Psaila JV, et al: Preparation of human saphenous vein for coronary artery bypass grafting impairs its capacity to produce prostacyclin. *Cardiovasc Res* 21:28–33, 1987.
31. Angelini GD, Christie M, Bryan AJ, et al: Preparation of human saphenous vein for coronary artery bypass grafting impairs its capacity to release endothelium derived relaxant factor. *Ann Thorac Surg* 48:417–420, 1989b.
32. Underwood MJ, More R, Weeraseena N, et al: The effect of surgical preparation and in vitro distension on the intrinsic fibrinolytic activity of human saphenous vein. *Eur J Vasc Surg* 7:518–522, 1993.
33. Roth G: Platelet arachidonate metabolism and platelet activating factor, in Shuman MA, Phillips DR (eds): *Biochemistry of Platelets.* New York/London, Academic Press, 1986, pp 69–114.
34. Jang IK, Fuster V: Mechanisms of plaque formation and occlusion in venous coronary bypass grafts, in Luscher T, Turina M, Braunwald E (eds): *Coronary Artery Graft Disease: Mechanisms and Prevention.* Berlin, Springer-Verlag, 1994, pp 42–52.
35. Lam JYT, Chesebro JH, Steele PM, et al: Vasospasm related to platelet deposition? Relationship in a porcine preparation of arterial injury in vivo. *Circulation* 75:243–248, 1987.
36. Fuster V, Chesebro JH: Aortocoronary artery vein graft disease: Experimental and clinical approach for the understanding of the role of platelets and platelet inhibitors. *Circulation* 72:V-65s–V-70s, 1985.
37. Davies MG, Klyachkin ML, Dalen H, et al: The integrity of experimental vein graft endothelium: Implications on the etiology of early graft failure. *Eur J Vasc Surg* 7:156–165, 1993.
38. Newby AC, George SJ: Proposed roles for growth factors in mediating

smooth muscle cell proliferation in vascular pathologies. *Cardiovasc Res* 27:1173–1183, 1993.

39. Jawien A, Bowen-Pope DF, Lindner V, et al: Platelet-derived growth factor promotes smooth muscle cell migration and intimal thickening in a rat model of balloon angioplasty. *J Clin Invest* 89:507–511, 1992.
40. Bornfeldt KE, Raines EW, Nakano T, et al: Insulin-like growth factor and platelet-derived growth factor BB induce directed migration of human arterial smooth muscle cells via signalling pathways that are distinct from those of proliferation. *J Clin Invest* 93:1266–1274, 1994.
41. Nabel EG, Yang Z, Liptay S, et al: Recombinant platelet derived growth factor B gene expression in porcine arteries induce intimal hyperplasia in vivo. *J Clin Invest* 91:1822–1829, 1993.
42. Francis SE, Hunter S, Holt CM, et al: Release of platelet-derived growth factor activity from arteriovenous bypass grafts. *J Thorac Cardiovasc Surg* 108:540–548, 1994.
43. Hughes S, Hall PA: Overview of the fibroblast growth factor and receptor families: Complexity, functional diversity, and implications for future cardiovascular research. *Cardiovasc Res* 27:1199–1203, 1993.
44. Lindner V, Lappi DA, Baird A, et al: Role of basic fibroblast growth factor in vascular lesion formation. *Circ Res* 68:106–113, 1991.
45. Edelmann ER, Nugent MA, Smith LT, et al: Basic fibroblast growth factor enhances the coupling of intimal hyperplasia and proliferation of *vasa vasorum* in injured rat arteries. *J Clin Invest* 89:465–473, 1992.
46. Olson NE, Chao S, Lindner V, et al: Intimal smooth muscle cell proliferation after balloon injury: The role of basic fibroblast growth factor. *Am J Pathol* 140:1017–1023, 1992.
47. Nabel EG, Yang Z, Plautz G, et al: Recombinant fibroblast growth factor-1 promotes intimal hyperplasia and angiogenesis in arteries in vivo. *Nature* 362:844–846, 1993.
48. Lindner V, Reidy MA: Expression of basic fibroblast growth factor and its receptor by smooth muscle cells and endothelium in injured rat arteries: An en face study. *Circ Res* 73:589–595, 1993.
49. Sidawy AN, Hakim FS, Neville RF, et al: Autoradiographic mapping and characterization of insulin like growth factor-1 receptor binding in human greater saphenous vein. *J Vasc Surg* 18:947–953, 1993.
50. Miano JM, Tota RR, Vlasic N, et al: Early proto-oncogene expression in rat aortic smooth muscle cells following endothelial removal. *Am J Pathol* 137:761–765, 1990.
51. Bauters C, de Groote P, Adamantidis M, et al: Proto-oncogene expression in rabbit aorta after wall injury: First marker of the cellular process leading to restenosis after angioplasty? *Eur Heart J* 13:556–559, 1992.
52. Moggio RA, Ding J-Z, Smith CJ, et al: Immediate early gene expression in human saphenous veins harvested during coronary bypass graft operations. *J Thorac Cardiovasc Surg* 110:209–213, 1995.
53. Quist WC, Haudenschild CC, LoGerfo FW: Qualitative microscopy of

implanted vein grafts: Effects of graft integrity on morphologic fate. *J Thorac Cardiovasc Surg* 103:671–677, 1992.
54. Clowes AW, Reidy MA, Clowes MM: Kinetics of cellular proliferation after arterial injury: I. Smooth muscle cell growth in the absence of endothelium. *Lab Invest* 49:327–333, 1983.
55. Friedman RJ, Stemerman MB, Wenz B, et al: The effect of thrombocytopenia on experimental atherosclerotic lesion formation in rabbit. *J Clin Invest* 60:1191–1201, 1977.
56. Angelini GD: Saphenous vein graft failure: Etiologic considerations and strategies for prevention. *Curr Opin Cardiol* 7:939–944, 1992.
57. Hedin U, Thyberg J: Plasma fibronectin promotes modulation of arterial smooth muscle cells from contractile to synthetic phenotype. *Differentiation* 33:239–246, 1987.
58. Madri JA, Kocher O, Merwin JR, et al: The interactions of vascular cells with solid phase (matrix) and soluble factors. *J Cardiovasc Pharmacol* 14:70S–75S, 1989.
59. Zempo N, Kenagy RD, Au YPT, et al: Matrix metalloproteinases of vascular wall cells are increased in balloon-injured rat carotid artery. *J Vasc Surg* 20:209–217, 1994.
60. Southgate KM, Izzat MB, Knight D, et al: Upregulation of matrix degrading gelatinases in pig saphenous vein grafts. *Br Heart J* 75:P46S, 1995.
61. Angelini GD, Newby AC: The future of saphenous vein as a coronary artery bypass conduit. *Eur Heart J* 10:273–280, 1989.
62. Yang Z, Luscher TF: Basic cellular mechanisms of coronary bypass graft disease. *Eur Heart J* 14:193S–197S, 1993.
63. Luscher TF, Yang Z, Oemar BS: Endothelium and vascular smooth muscle function of coronary bypass grafts, in Luscher TF, Turina M, Braunwald E (eds): *Coronary Artery Graft Disease: Mechanisms and Prevention.* Berlin, Springer-Verlag, 1994, pp 193–212.
64. Davies AH, Magee TR, Baird RN, et al: Vein compliance: A preoperative indicator of vein morphology and of veins at risk of vascular graft stenosis. *Br J Surg* 79:1019–1021, 1992.
65. Panetta TF, Marin ML, Veith FJ, et al: Unsuspected preexisting saphenous vein disease: An unrecognised cause of vein bypass failure. *J Vasc Surg* 15:102–112, 1992.
66. Marin ML, Veith FJ, Panetta TF, et al: Saphenous vein biopsy: A predictor of vein graft failure. *J Vasc Surg* 18:407–415, 1993.
67. Chan P, Munro E, Patel M, et al: Cellular biology of human intimal hyperplastic stenosis. *Eur J Vasc Surg* 7:129–135, 1993.
68. Chan P, Patel M, Betteridge L, et al: Abnormal growth regulation of vascular smooth muscle cells by heparin in patients with restenosis. *Lancet* 341:341–342, 1993.
69. Stonebridge PA, Miller A, Tsooskas AL, et al: Angioscopy of arm vein infrainguinal bypass grafts. *Ann Vasc Surg* 5:170–175, 1991.
70. Zilla P, von Oppell U, Deutsch M: The endothelium: A key to the future. *J Card Surg* 8:32–60, 1993.

71. Davies MG, Hagen P-O: Pathophysiology of vein graft failure: A review. *Eur J Vasc Endovasc Surg* 9:7–18, 1995.
72. Ramos JR, Berger K, Mansfield PB, et al: Histological fate and endothelial changes of distended and non-distended vein grafts. *Ann Surg* 183:205–228, 1976.
73. Gundry SR, Jones M, Ishihara T, et al: Optimal preparation techniques for human saphenous vein grafts. *Surgery* 88:785–794, 1980.
74. LoGerfo FW, Quist WC, Cantelmo ML, et al: Integrity of vein grafts as a function of intimal and medial preservation. *Circulation* 68:II–117S–II–124S, 1983.
75. Angelini GD, Breckenridge IM, Butchart EG, et al: Metabolic damge to human saphenous vein during preparation for coronary artery bypass grafting. *Cardiovasc Res* 19:326–334, 1985.
76. Angelini GD, Passani SL, Breckenridge IM, et al: Nature and pressure dependence of damage induced by distension of human saphenous vein coronary artery bypass grafts. *Cardiovasc Res* 21:902–907, 1987.
77. Soyombo AA, Angelini GD, Bryan AJ, et al: Surgical preparation induces injury and promotes smooth muscle cell proliferation in a culture of human saphenous vein. *Cardiovasc Res* 27:1961–1967, 1993.
78. Soyombo AA, Angelini GD, Newby AC: Neointima formation is promoted by surgical preparation and inhibited by cyclic nucleotides in human saphenous vein organ cultures. *J Thorac Cardiovasc Surg* 109:2–12, 1995.
79. O'Neil G, Chester AH, Schyns CJ, et al: Effect of surgical preparation and arterialization on vasomotion of human saphenous vein. *J Thorac Cardiovasc Surg* 107:699–706, 1994.
80. Zwolak RM, Adams MC, Clowes AW: Kinetics of vein graft hyperplasia: Association with tangential stress. *J Vasc Surg* 5:126–136, 1987.
81. Schwartz LB, O'Donohue MK, Purut CM, et al: Myointimal thickening in experimental vein grafts is dependent on wall tension. *J Vasc Surg* 15:176–186, 1992.
82. Galt SW, Zwolak RM, Wagner RJ, et al: Differential responses of arteries and vein grafts to blood flow reduction. *J Vasc Surg* 17:563–570, 1993.
83. Dobrin PB: On the roles of deformation, tension, and wall stress as critical stimuli eliciting myointimal/medial hyperplasia. *J Vasc Surg* 15:581–582, 1992.
84. Hsieh H-J, Li N-Q, Frangos JA: Shear stress induced platelet-derived growth factor gene expression in human endothelial cells is mediated by protein kinase C. *J Cell Physiol* 150:552–558, 1992.
85. Sterpetti AV, Cucina A, Fragale A, et al: Shear stress influences the release of platelet-derived growth factor and basic fibroblast growth factor by arterial smooth muscle cells. *Eur J Vasc Surg* 8:138–142, 1994.
86. Rubanyi GM, Freay AD, Kauser K, et al: Mechanoreception by the endothelium: Mediators and mechanisms of pressure and flow induced vascular responses. *Blood Vessels* 27:246–257, 1990.

87. Costa KA, Sumpio BE, Cerreta JM: Increased elastin synthesis by cultured bovine aortic smooth muscle cells subjected to repetitive mechanical stretching. *FASEB J* 5:1609A, 1991.
88. Sumpio BE, Banes AJ: Response of porcine aortic smooth muscle cells to cyclic tensional deformation. *J Surg Res* 44:696–701, 1988.
89. Chaikhouni A, Crawford FA, Kochel PJ, et al: Human internal mammary artery produces more prostacyclin than saphenous vein. *J Thorac Cardiovasc Surg* 92:88–91, 1986.
90. Luscher TF, Diederich D, Siebenmann R, et al: Difference between endothelium-dependent relaxations in arterial and in venous coronary bypass grafts. *N Engl J Med* 319:462–467, 1988.
91. Sala A, Rona P, Pompilio G, et al: Prostacylcin production by different human grafts employed in coronary operations. *Ann Thorac Surg* 57:1147–1150, 1994.
92. He G-W, Ryan WH, Acuff TE, et al: Greater contractility of internal mammary artery bifurcation: Possible cause of low patency rates. *Ann Thorac Surg* 58:529–532, 1994.
93. Morin JE, Hedderich G, Poirier NL, et al: Coronary artery bypass using internal mammary artery branches. *Ann Thorac Surg* 54:911–914, 1992.
94. Predel HG, Yang Z, Von Segesser L, et al: Implications of pulsatile stretch on growth of saphenous vein and mammary artery smooth muscle. *Lancet* 340:878–879, 1992.
95. Holt CM, Francis SE, Newby AC, et al: Comparison of responses to injury in organ culture of human saphenous vein and internal mammary artery. *Ann Thorac Surg* 55:1522–1528, 1993.
96. Nguyen HC, Grossi EA, LeBoutillier M, et al: Mammary artery versus saphenous vein grafts: Assessment of basic fibroblast growth factor receptors. *Ann Thorac Surg* 58:308–311, 1994.
97. Van Son JA, Smedts F, Vincent JG, et al: Comparative anatomic studies of various arterial conduits for myocardial revascularization. *J Thorac Cardiovasc Surg* 99:703–707, 1990.
98. He G-W, Yang C-Q: Comparison between arterial grafts and coronary artery: An attempt at functional classification. *J Thorac Cardiovasc Surg* 109:707–715, 1995.
99. Van Son JAM, Smedts F, de Wilde PCM, et al: Histological study of the internal mammary artery with emphasis on its suitability as a coronary artery bypass graft. *Ann Thorac Surg* 55:106–113, 1993.
100. Bach RG, Kern MJ, Donohue TJ, et al: Comparison of phasic blood flow velocity characteristics of arterial and venous coronary artery bypass conduits. *Circulation* 88(pt 2):133–140, 1993.
101. Louagie YAG, Haxhe J-P, Buche M, et al: Intraoperative electromagnetic flowmeter measurements in coronary artery bypass grafts. *Ann Thorac Surg* 57:357–364, 1994.
102. Loop FD, Thomas JD: Hypoperfusion after arterial bypass grafting. *Ann Thorac Surg* 56:812–813, 1993.
103. Vajtai P, Ravichandran PS, Fessler CL, et al: Inadequate internal mam-

mary artery graft as a cause of postoperative ischemia: Diagnosis and management. *Eur J Cardiothorac Surg* 6:603–608, 1992.

104. Navia D, Cosgrove DM, Lytle BW, et al: Is the internal thoracic artery the conduit of choice to replace a stenotic vein graft? *Ann Thorac Surg* 57:40–44, 1994.
105. Hanet C, Schroeder E, Michel X, et al: Flow-induced vasomotor response to tachycardia of the human internal mammary artery and saphenous vein grafts late following bypass surgery. *Circulation* 84:III-268S–III-274S, 1991.
106. Kushwaha SS, Bustami M, Tadjkarimi S, et al: Late endothelial function of free and pedicled internal mammary artery grafts. *J Thorac Cardiovasc* 110:453–462, 1995.
107. Chester AH, Yacoub MH: Biological and vasomotor properties of the gastroepiploic and inferior epigastric arteries, in Angelini GD, Bryan AJ, Dion R (eds): *Arterial Conduits in Myocardial Revascularisation.* London, Edward Arnold, 1995, pp 32–37.
108. Lytle BW, Loop FD, Cosgrove DM, et al: Long-term (5 to 12 years) serial studies of internal mammary artery and saphenous vein coronary bypass grafts. *J Thorac Cardiovasc Surg* 89:248–258, 1985.
109. Bernal JM, Rabasa JM, Echevarria JR, et al: A multivariate analysis of factors affecting early coronary artery bypass patency. *Coron Artery Dis* 2:713–716, 1991.
110. Roth JA, Cukingnan RA, Brown BG, et al: Factors influencing patency of saphenous vein grafts. *Ann Thorac Surg* 28:1976–1980, 1979.
111. Cataldo G, Braga M, Pirotta N, et al: Factors influencing 1-year patency of coronary artery saphenous vein grafts. *Circulation* 1993, 88:II-93S–II-98S, 1993.
112. Paz MA, Lupon J, Bosch X, et al: Predictors of early saphenous vein aortocoronary bypass graft occlusion. *Ann Thorac Surg* 56:1101–1106, 1993.
113. O'Connor GT, Plume SK, Olmstead EM, et al: A regional prospective study on in-hospital mortality associated with coronary artery bypass grafting. *JAMA* 266:803–809, 1991.
114. Hannan EL, O'Donnell JF, Kilburn H Jr, et al: Investigation of the relationship between volume and mortality for surgical procedures performed in New York state hospitals. *JAMA* 262:503–510, 1989.
115. Bex JP, Latini L, Durandy Y: The art of cardiac surgery: Critical analysis of the limits of statistics in cardiac surgery. *J Cardiac Surg* 9:288–291, 1994.
116. Perrault LP, Carrier M, Hebert Y, et al: Early experience with the inferior epigastric artery in coronary artery bypass grafting. *J Thorac Cardiovasc Surg* 106:928–930, 1993.
117. Buche M, Schroeder E, Gurne O, et al: Coronary artery bypass grafting with the inferior epigastric artery: Midterm clinical and angiographic results. *J Thorac Cardiovasc Surg* 109:553–560, 1995.
118. Boerboom LE, Olinger GO, Bonchek LI, et al: The relative influence of arterial pressure versus intra-operative distention on lipid accumu-

lation in primate vein bypass grafts. *J Thorac Cardiovasc Surg* 90:756–764, 1985.

119. Klyachkin ML, Davies MG, Svendsen E, et al: Hypercholesterolemia and experimental vein grafts: Accelerated development of intimal hyperplasia and abnormal vasomotor function. *J Surg Res* 54:451–468, 1993.
120. Campeau L, Enjalbert M, Lesperance J, et al: The relationship of risk factors to the development of atherosclerosis in saphenous vein bypass grafts and the progression of disease in the native circulation: A study 10 years after aorotocoronary bypass surgery. *N Engl J Med* 311:1329–1332, 1984.
121. Hoff HF, Beck GJ, Skibinski CI, et al: Serum Lp[a] level as a predictor of vein graft stenosis after coronary artery bypass surgery in patients. *Circulation* 77:1238–1244, 1988.
122. Simpson HCR, Meade TW, Stirling Y, et al: Hypertriglyceridemia and hypercoagulability. *Lancet* I:786–789, 1983.
123. Drexel H, Amann FW: Lipids and lipid lowering drugs and graft function, in Luscher T, Turina M, Braunwald E (eds): *Coronary Artery Graft Disease: Mechanisms and Prevention.* Berlin, Springer Verlag, 1994, pp 247–258.
124. Lawrie GM, Morris GC, Earle N: Long-term results of coronary bypass surgery. *Ann Surg* 213:377–387, 1991.
125. Solymoss BC, Nadeau P, Millette D, et al: Late thrombosis of saphenous vein coronary bypass grafts related to risk factors. *Circulation* 78:I-140s–I-144s, 1988.
126. Lehmann KH, von Segesser L, Muller-Glauser W, et al: Internal mammary coronary artery grafts: Is their superiority also due to a basically intact endothelium. *Thorac Cardiovasc Surg* 37:187–189, 1989.
127. Lehtola A, Verkkala K, Jarvinen A: Is electrocautery safe for internal mammary artery mobilization? A study using scanning electron microscopy. *Thorac Cardiovasc Surg* 37:55–57, 1989.
128. Johns RA, Peach MJ, Flanagan T, et al: Probing of the canine mammary artery damages endothelium and impairs vasodilation resulting from prostacyclin and endothelium-derived relaxing factor. *J Thorac Cardiovasc Surg* 97:252–258, 1989.
129. Cooper GJ, Gillot R, Francis SE, et al: Distension produces medial but not endothelial damage in porcine internal mammary artery. *Cardiovasc Surg* 3:171–174, 1995.
130. Treasure T: Damage to an internal mammary artery graft at dissection. *Br Heart J* 70:390, 1993.
131. Dougenis D, Robinson MC, Brown AH: Acute dissection of the internal mammary artery: A fatal complication of coronary artery bypass grafting. *J Cardiovasc Surg (Torino)* 31:589–591, 1990.
132. Goldman S, Copeland J, Moritz T, et al: Internal mammary artery and saphenous vein graft patency: Effects of aspirin. *Circulation* 82:IV-237S–IV-242S, 1990.
133. Bonchek LE: Prevention of endothelial damage during preparation of

saphenous veins for bypass grafting. *J Thorac Cardiovasc Surg* 79:911–915, 1980.

134. LoGerfo FW, Quist WC, Crawshaw JM, et al: An improved technique for preservation of endothelial morphology in vein grafts. *Surgery* 90:1015–1024, 1981.
135. Angelini GD, Breckenridge IM, Williams HM, et al: A surgical preparative technique for coronary bypass grafts of human saphenous vein which preserves medial and endothelial functional integrity. *J Thorac Cardiovasc Surg* 94:393–398, 1987.
136. He G-W, Rosenfeldt FL, Angus JA: Pharmacologic relaxation of the saphenous vein during harvesting for coronary artery bypass grafting. *Ann Thorac Surg* 55:1210–1217, 1993.
137. Angelini GD, Bryan AJ, Hunter S, et al: A simple technique for preservation of saphenous vein integrity during coronary artery bypass grafting. *Ann Thorac Surg* 53:871–874, 1992.
138. Waters DJ, Thomsen TA: Saphenous vein preparation for coronary artery bypass grafting using a cardioplegia delivery set. *Ann Thorac Surg* 56:385–386, 1993.
139. Chesebro JH, Clements IP, Fuster V, et al: A platelet inhibitor drug trial in coronary artery bypass operations: Benefit of perioperative dipyridamole and aspirin therapy on early postoperative vein graft patency. *N Engl J Med* 307:73–78, 1982.
140. Israel DH, Adams PC, Stein B, et al: Antithrombotic therapy in the coronary vein graft patient. *Clin Cardiol* 14:283–295, 1991.
141. Fremes SE, Levinton C, Naylor CD, et al: Optimal antithrombotic therapy following aortocoronary bypass: A meta-analysis. *Eur J Cardiothorac Surg* 7:169–180, 1993.
142. Antiplatelet Trialists' Collaboration: Collaborative overview of randomised trials of antiplatelet therapy: II. Maintenance of vascular graft or arterial patency by antiplatelet therapy. *BMJ* 308:159–168, 1994.
143. Rajah SM, Nair U, Rees M, et al: Effects of antiplatelet therapy with indobufen or aspirin-dipyridamole on graft patency one year after coronary artery bypass grafting. *J Thorac Cardiovasc Surg* 107:1146–1153, 1994.
144. Van Der Meer J, Hillege HL, Kootstra GJ, et al: Prevention of one year vein graft occlusion after aortocoronary bypass surgery: A comparison of low dose aspirin, low dose aspirin plus dipyridamole, and oral anticoagulants. *Lancet* 342:257–264, 1993.
145. Pfisterer M, Burkart F, Jockers G, et al: Trial of low-dose aspirin plus dipyridamole versus anticoagulants for prevention of aortocoronary vein graft occlusion. *Lancet* II:1–6, 1989.
146. Weber MAJ, Hasford J, Taillens C, et al: Low dose aspirin versus anticoagulants for prevention of coronary graft occlusion. *Am J Cardiol* 66:1464–1468, 1990.
147. Goldman S, Copeland J, Mortiz T, et al: Long term graft patency (3 years) after coronary artery surgery. Effects of aspirin: Results of a VA Cooperative Study. *Circulation* 89:1138–1143, 1994.

148. Fuster V, Dyken ML, Vokonas PS, et al: Aspirin as a therapeutic agent in cardiovascular disease.. *Circulation* 37:659–675, 1993.
149. Antiplatelet Trialists' Collaboration: Collaborative overview of randomised trials of antiplatelet therapy: I. Prevention of death, myocardial infarction and stroke by prolonged antiplatelet therapy in various categories of patients. *BMJ* 308:81–106, 1994.
150. Clowes AW, Reidy MA: Prevention of stenosis after vascular reconstruction: Pharmacologic control of intimal hyperplasia: A review. *J Vasc Surg* 13:885–891, 1991.
151. Francis SE, Holt CM, Taylor T, et al: Heparin and myointimal thickening in an organ culture of human saphenous vein. *Atherosclerosis* 93:155–156, 1992.
152. Cambria RP, Ivarsson BL, Fallon JT, et al: Heparin fails to suppress intimal proliferation in experimental vein grafts. *Surgery* 111:424–429, 1992.
153. Ellis SG, Roubin GS, Wilentz J, et al: Effect of 18 to 24 hour heparin administration for prevention of restenosis after uncomplicated coronary angioplasty. *Am Heart J* 117:777–782, 1989.
154. Edmondson RA, Cohen AT, Das SK, et al: Low-molecular weight heparin versus aspirin and dipyridamole after femoropopliteal bypass grafting. *Lancet* 344:914–918, 1994.
155. Gottlieb SO: Calcium antagonists in patients undergoing coronary artery byapss surgery, in Luscher TF, Turina Mk, Braunwald E (eds): *Coronary Artery Graft Disease: Mechanisms and Prevention.* Berlin, Springer-Verlag, 1994, pp 312–327.
156. Yang Z, Noll G, Luscher TF: Calcium antagonists differently inhibit proliferation of human coronary smooth muscle cells in response to pulsatile stretch and platelet-derived growth factor. *Circulation* 88:832–836, 1993.
157. Emanuelsson H, Beatt KJ, Bagger J-P, et al: Long term effects of angiopeptin treatment in coronary angioplasty: Reduction of clinical events but not angiographic restenosis. *Circulation* 91:1689–1696, 1995.
158. MERCATOR Study Group: Does the new angiotensin converting enzyme inhibitor cilazapril prevent restenosis after percutaneous transluminal coronary angioplasty? *Circulation* 86:100–110, 1992.
159. Kranzhofer R, Schirmer J, Schomig A, et al: Suppression of neointimal thickening and smooth muscle cell proliferation after arterial injury in the rat by inhibitors of Na^+-H^+ exchange. *Circ Res* 73:264–268, 1993.
160. Mitsuka M, Nagae M, Berk B: Na^+-H^+ exchange inhibitors decrease neointimal formation after rat carotid injury. *Circ Res* 73:269–275, 1993.
161. Blankenhorn DH, Nessim SA, Johnson RL, et al: Beneficial effect of combined colestipol-niacin therapy on coronary atherosclerosis and coronary venous bypass grafts. *JAMA* 257:3233–3240, 1987.
162. Cashin-Hemphill L, Mack WJ, Pogoda JM, et al: Beneficial effects of

colestipol-niacin on coronary atherosclerosis. *JAMA* 264:3013–3017, 1990.

163. Kohler TR, Kirkman TR, Clowes AW: The effect of rigid external support on vein graft adaptation to the arterial circulation. *J Vasc Surg* 9:277–285, 1989.
164. Batellier J, Wassef M, Merial R, et al: Protection from atherosclerosis in vein grafts by a rigid external support. *Arterioscler Thromb* 13:379–384, 1993.
165. Violaris AG, Newby AC, Angelini GD: Effects of external stenting on wall thickening in arteriovenous bypass grafts. *Ann Thorac Surg* 55:667–671, 1993.
166. Angelini GD, Izzat MB, Bryan AJ, et al: External stenting reduces medial and neointimal thickening in a pig model of arteriovenous bypass grafting. *J Thorac Cardiovasc Surg,* in press.
167. Izzat MB, Mehta D, Bryan AJ, et al: The influence of external stent size on early medial and neointimal thickening in a pig model of saphenous vein bypass grafting. *Circulation*, in press.
168. Nyamekye I, Anglin S, McEwan J, et al: Photodynamic therapy of normal and balloon-injured rat carotid arteries using 5-amino-levulinic acid. *Circulation* 91:417–425, 1995.
169. March KL, Patton BL, Wilensky RL, et al: 8-Methoxypsoralen and long wave ultraviolet irradiation: A novel, antiproliferative combination for vascular smooth muscle. *Circulation* 87:184–191, 1993.
170. LaMuraglia GM, Klyachkin ML, Adili F, et al: Photodynamic therapy of vein grafts: Suppression of intimal hyperplasia of the vein graft but not the anastomosis. *J Vasc Surg* 21:882–890, 1995.
171. Ferns GA, Raines EW, Sprugel KH, et al: Inhibition of neointimal smooth muscle accumulation after angioplasty by an antibody to PDGF. *Science* 253:1129–1132, 1991.
172. Lindner V, Reidy MA: Proliferation of smooth muscle cells after vascular injury is inhibited by an antibody against basic fibroblast growth factor. *Proc Natl Acad Sci U S A* 88:3739–3743, 1991.
173. Choi ET, Engel L, Callow AD, et al: Inhibition of neointimal hyperplasia by blocking $a_v b_3$ integrin with a small peptide fragment Gpen GRGDSPCA. *J Vasc Surg* 19:125–134, 1994.
174. More RS, Underwood MJ, de Bono DP: Targeting fibrinolytic agents to the vessel wall: A new therapeutic niche? *Thromb Haemost* 71:158–159, 1994.
175. Underwood MJ, Pringle SW, de Bono DP: Reduction of thrombus formation in vivo using a thrombolytic agent targeted at damaged endothelial cells. *Br J Surg* 79:915–917, 1992.
176. Dzau VJ, Pratt RE: Antisense technology to block autocrine growth factors. *J Vasc Surg* 15:934–935, 1992.
177. Simons M, Edelmann ER, DeKeyser J-L, et al: Antisense *c-myb* oligonucleotides inhibit arterial smooth muscle cell accumulation in vivo. *Nature* 359:67–70, 1992.

178. Bennett MR, Anglin S, McEwan JR, et al: Inhibition of vascular smooth muscle cell proliferation in vitro and in vivo by *c-myc* antisense oligonucleotides. *J Clin Invest* 93:820–828, 1994.
179. Simons M, Rosenberg RD: Antisense nonmuscle myosin heavy chain and *c-myb* oligonucleotides suppress smooth muscle cell proliferation in vitro. *Circulation* 70:835–843, 1992.
180. Shi Y, Hutchinson HG, Hall DJ, et al: Downregulation of *c-myc* expression by antisense oligonucleotides inhibits proliferation of human smooth muscle cells. *Circulation* 88:1190–1195, 1993.
181. Conte MS, Birinyi LK, Miyata T, et al: Efficient repopulation of denuded rabbit arteries with autologous genetically modified endothelial cells. *Circulation* 23:2161–2169, 1994.
182. Chen SJ, Wilson JM, Muller DWM: Adenovirus mediated gene transfer of soluble vascular adhesion molecule to porcine interposition vein grafts. *Circulation* 89:1922–1928, 1994.

Aortic Valve Sparing in Aortic Root Disease

Richard P. Cochran, M.D.
Associate Professor, Division of Cardiothoracic Surgery, University of Washington, Seattle

Karyn S. Kunzelman, Ph.D.
Research Assistant Professor, Division of Cardiothoracic Surgery; Adjunct Faculty, Center for Bioengineering, University of Washington, Seattle

In the past two decades, as surgical techniques have improved and the complications of prosthetic valves have been realized, "valve-sparing" operations have become increasingly more popular. The efforts and successes in valve sparing were initially seen in treatment of mitral and tricuspid valvular disease. During the past five years, however, there has been increased interest in valve-sparing procedures for the aortic valve, particularly in diseases that involve the "aortic root" as opposed to those that involve only the aortic valve. This tendency is logical, in that intrinsic aortic valve disease precludes the benefit of valve sparing. As such, most technical advances in this area have dealt with valve sparing in diseases that affect the aortic root as a composite structure. In this chapter, we discuss the currently available techniques for valve sparing in aortic root disease and their advantages and disadvantages. In addition, we present what we believe is the best of these techniques.

Aortic valve sparing is not a new concept. The techniques discussed in this chapter are the result of surgical innovation and biomechanical understanding and their interaction and evolution over many years. Because of this long evolution, however, there is significant variation, and often difference of opinion, regarding the anatomical terms and definitions that apply to this region of reconstruction known as the aortic root. In addition, many of the biomechanical concepts are not familiar to practicing surgeons. Some clarifications are necessary in both areas. Before we can begin a meaningful discussion of the exciting new developments in this area of cardiac surgery, some background information is necessary.

Advances in Cardiac Surgery®, vol. 8
© 1996, Mosby–Year Book, Inc.

ANATOMY

The aortic root has fascinated anatomists, physicians, and surgeons for centuries. Leonardo da Vinci illustrated the aortic root quite accurately as early as 1513.[1] Although the term aortic root is familiar and well understood, it is not defined in either *Stedman's Dictionary*[2] or *Dorland's Dictionary.*[3] Nor is it addressed in *Gray's Anatomy*[4] or *Grant's Atlas of Anatomy.*[5] Fortunately, this lack of formal definition has not prevented the tremendous strides made during the past two decades in surgical treatment of aortic root disease. The vagueness in terminology, however, does require that some definitions be established before a discussion of surgical interventions can proceed. For this chapter, the aortic root is defined as the region that begins at the left ventricular outflow tract, at what we agree is the aortic "annulus" (Fig 1). The annulus is one of the controversial aspects of the aortic root, and there is disagreement among anatomists and surgeons regarding the correct area to be so termed. In fact, some argue that no true annulus exists. However, because any aortic reconstruction must involve the origin of the aorta, and the origin has been traditionally called the annulus, the term will be used. For this discussion, we favor the subvalvular aortic annulus described by anatomists. This defines the annulus as a circular orifice,[4] not as a crown-shaped annulus described by some surgeons.[6] Distal to the annulus, the aortic root includes the aortic valve leaflets, the aortic wall, the sinuses of Valsalva, and the coronary ostia. The aortic root terminates just distal to these structures at the sinotubular junction. The portion of the aorta just distal to the sinotubular junction is considered the ascending aorta. These definitions of the aortic root are chosen to help address the complex interactions that occur in this region, as well as to help tailor surgical interventions that best recreate normal anatomy.

Although at first glance the aortic root appears relatively

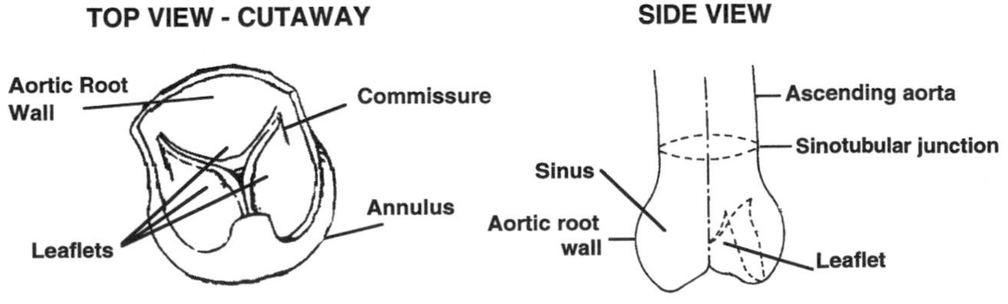

FIGURE 1.
Schematic representation of aortic root components.

simple in structural sense, it is in reality a complex geometric structure with balanced biomechanical interactions that are just beginning to be fully understood. This complex biomechanical structure accomplishes many functions. It is the interaction of all root components that maintains forward blood flow from the left ventricle and ensures coronary perfusion. In addition, the resultant biomechanical forces are balanced in a manner that makes the aortic root efficient and durable. The complex biomechanical interactions of the aortic root are both its strength and its potential weakness. Disruption of any geometric component of the aortic root affects all other components and can alter the biomechanics of the whole system. Unfortunately, several disease processes can and do alter the geometry.

This interaction and interdependence of the aortic root is just now being fully understood. Before this concept of interdependence in the aortic root was developed, diseases were viewed as originating from the structural component that ultimately failed, not from the components that started the disruption of the interaction. Because geometric disruption of any root component may alter valve function, all aortic root problems were historically presumed to be valve related. This simplistic approach has recently been questioned. Regarding all aortic root problems as valve related oversimplified the problem and delayed understanding of the complex interaction of the components; thus, the development of appropriate surgical intervention was delayed. Surgical techniques for valve sparing now acknowledge this previous oversimplification. Understanding the biomechanics of the aortic root is necessary for surgeons to become more adept at addressing this once formidable anatomical region.

BIOMECHANICS

The normal aortic root carries out its biomechanical functions very efficiently and with great durability. A complex biomechanical system of stress sharing allows the aortic root to tolerate large changes in pressure and significant alterations in stress during the cardiac cycle, as well as to accommodate a fair amount of pathologic alteration. The critical mechanical components of the aortic root include a physiologically appropriate annulus, a valve with pliable leaflets, sinuses of Valsalva of appropriate depth, and a well-formed sinotubular junction. These components all work in concert to accomplish the roles of the aortic root. The composite functional outcome of their interaction is creation of eddy formations within the flowing blood during ventricular ejection. These eddy formations aid in valve closure and ensure coronary ostial perfusion (Fig 2). In addition to physiologic benefit from the aortic root configuration, there is mechanical benefit from the curvilinear attachment between the aortic valve leaflets and aortic root wall. This arrangement allows high stresses carried by each leaflet during closure to be shared with the aortic root wall (Fig 3). Further mechanical benefit is realized in this interactive system, in that appropriate valve closure and leaflet coaptation allow for compressive support for each leaflet from its adjacent leaflets, thereby reducing tensile stresses in each individual leaflet. Although simple in appearance at first glance, this complex biomechanical system has proved difficult to simulate. As such, a more simplified view of the aortic root was historically adopted for surgical intervention. This simplification allowed interventions to begin where previ-

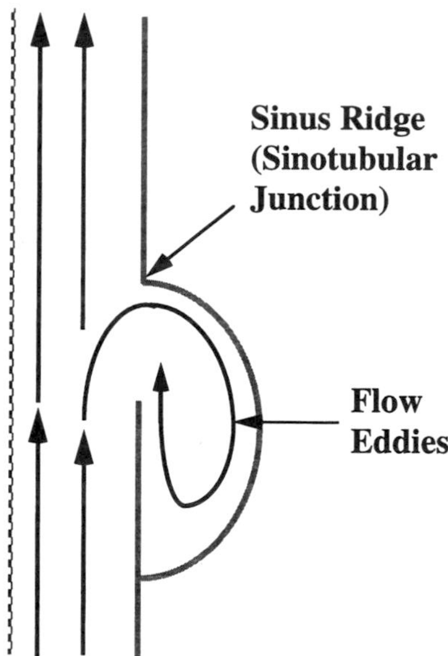

FIGURE 2.
Schematic representation of aortic valve and root demonstrating the role of the sinus ridge in the creation of eddy currents for enhanced valve closure and coronary perfusion. (Courtesy of Cochran RP, Kunzelman KS, Eddy AC, et al: Modified conduit preparation creates a pseudosinus in an aortic valve sparing procedure for aneurysm of the ascending aorta. *J Thoracic Cardiovascular Surg* 109:1049–1058, 1995.)

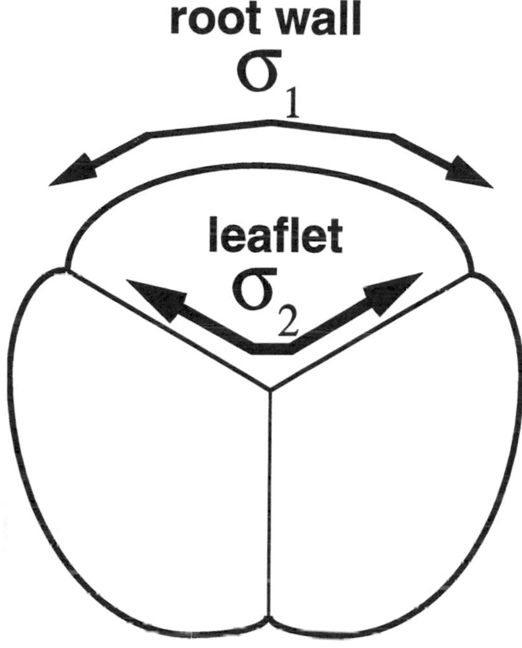

FIGURE 3.
Schematic representation of stress in leaflets and root wall. Because the leaflets are thinner, the stresses will be higher than in the root wall. The curvilinear attachment at the sinuses, however, allows the high stress to be partially transferred to the root wall, thus decreasing the stress on the leaflets.

ously none had existed. Unfortunately, the simplified approach also created some misunderstanding and may have actually slowed the evolution toward a more anatomically and physiologically appropriate surgical approach.

HISTORICAL PERSPECTIVE

Historically, cardiac surgery developed as an operative effort to treat disease processes that were considered fatal if the abnormality was not corrected. As such, early developments for correction of cardiac abnormalities were directed at expedient and reproducible operative techniques. Unfortunately, not all life-threatening problems lent themselves to expedient surgical interventions. Two areas in which expeditious solutions were not readily available involved aortic root problems: aneurysms and dissections. As a result, evolution of therapeutic intervention for aortic root problems often followed divergent routes.

One technique that was developed to provide an expedient solution for aortic root problems was the Bentall procedure.[7] Although this procedure did offer expedience, both geometric and anatomical accuracy were sacrificed. In addition, this technique included a prosthetic valve; the associated complications were, most notably, thromboembolism and anticoagulation.[8–10] These complications have previously been described as "simply the exchange of one disease for another"[11] when a diseased valve is replaced. With this definition, in cases of dissection or aneurysm where an anatomically normal aortic valve may be involved, valvular replacement may be viewed as introduction of a new disease where formerly none existed.

Because of these concerns with prosthetic complications, resuspension of the aortic valve was described early in surgical treatment of ascending aortic dissections. These early efforts at valve sparing in dissection proved successful in both the short and long term, which opened the conceptual window for valve sparing in other aortic root processes, particularly aneurysm. Before extensive valve sparing could be undertaken, however, advances in other aspects of surgical intervention were necessary.

Concurrent to the efforts of valve resuspension in dissections, the field of cardiac surgery was rapidly advancing. Advances were made in surgical technique, materials technology, and surgical and medical management. These advances made extensive aortic root reconstruction and complex aortic valve–sparing procedures a possibility. Advances in surgical technique included refinement of valve suspension techniques, such as homograft and autograft placement. In addition to these technical advancements, a better understanding of the aortic root, its biomechanics, and its disease processes was gained. Materials technology improved to produce nonporous conduits. These conduits offer several advantages. They eliminate additional time for preclotting and reduce bleeding complications, both of which result in shortened operative time. Probably the most notable improvements occurred in surgical and medical management. Significant areas of improvement included myocardial protection, cardiopulmonary bypass, cardiac anesthesia, and coagulation management. Each of these advancements has made longer and more complex procedures more tolerable. As a result of the advances in these three areas, reparative surgery for the aortic valve has evolved to a new level and should now be considered a viable alternative to replacement. This evolution of reparative surgery for the aortic valve is similar to the evolution of mitral valve repair techniques, except that it occurred a decade later. Aortic valve sparing is becoming the procedure of choice for many diseases of the root, which had formerly included valve replacement as a component. The remainder of this chapter therefore deals with the valvular dilemma of the 1990s, which is when and how the aortic valve should be spared.

TECHNIQUES OF AORTIC VALVE–SPARING OPERATIONS FOR DISEASES OF THE AORTIC ROOT

As alluded to previously, there has been an evolution of aortic valve–sparing techniques. The techniques will probably evolve further, particularly as improvements in surgical technique, materials technology, and surgical and medical management continue. Each technique described in this chapter has been part of this evolutionary process. We first review the rationale and surgical approach of each technique and evaluate the strengths and weaknesses of each. We then describe in detail how aortic valve sparing with pseudosinus creation is done and why we think it the best anatomical and physiologic solution for these patients.

VALVE RESUSPENSION FOR AORTIC DISSECTIONS

Rationale

Aortic valve regurgitation caused by leaflet prolapse is a well recognized complication of aortic dissection and constitutes a major cause of morbidity and mortality if uncorrected in these patients. Successful surgical treatment of commissural disruption and leaflet prolapse in patients who have aortic dissection was reported as early as the 1960s.[12] Two trends emerged in the surgical treatment of these patients. The first technique, popular for speed and reproducibility, was replacement of the aortic root with a composite tube graft and aortic valve.[13–15] The second technique required more technical judgment in that it coupled preservation (resuspension) of the native aortic valve with repair of the dissection.[16–18] These early efforts at valve sparing were the first acknowledgment that composite replacement sacrificed a normal valve when treating aortic wall abnormalities.

Technique

Although there was substantial variability in the techniques used, the general operative approach was the same. The dissected ascending aorta was resected and replaced with a tubular graft (Fig 4). The technical challenge of the procedure was valve resuspension. Valve resuspension in a dissected aorta required obliteration of the false lumen and appropriate repositioning (resuspension) of

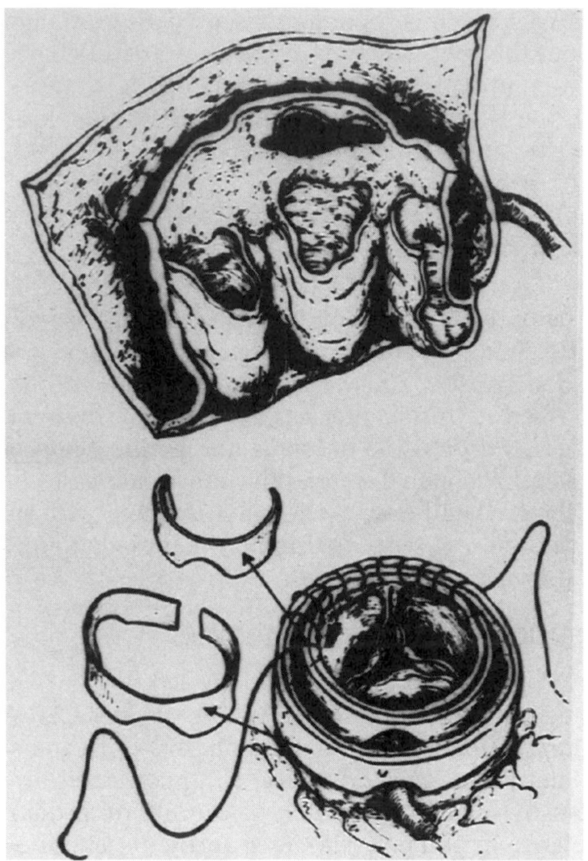

FIGURE 4.

Key components of valve resuspension for aortic dissection. Teflon felt is inserted in the false lumen, and the aortic valve is resuspended. (Courtesy of Miller DC: Surgical management of acute aortic dissection: New data. *Semin Thorac Cardiovasc Surg* 3:225–237, 1991.)

the disrupted valve commissures. An additional aspect that limited use of this technique was the recreation of the sinuses of Valsalva. When more than one commissure is disrupted, the sinuses of Valsalva are also disrupted, and appropriate valve sparing necessitates sinus reconstruction as well as commissural repositioning. The challenge of resuspension of one, two, or three of the aortic commissural posts in an appropriate orientation and the reconstruction of one or more sinuses of Valsalva were the limiting factors to wide acceptance of this very appealing procedure.

small button of arterial wall attached to the coronary ostia (Fig 5). Sutures are then placed from inside to outside the left ventricular outflow tract, immediately below the valve, at the level of the annulus. A Dacron graft is sized and then trimmed to remove a scalloped segment, which corresponds to the commissural post between the right and left leaflets. The previously placed subvalvular, or "annular" sutures are passed through the end of graft to correct the annular dilatation by fixing the size of the annulus to the size of the tube graft. The graft is then cut to 2–3 cm above the commissures, and the valve is resuspended within the graft, similar to valve resuspension or freehand homograft techniques. David et al.[20] have recently reported several modifications to this technique. These modifications do not include subvalvular stitch placement. Rather the sinuses are excised and reconstructed selectively, such that remodeling of the sinuses may be addressed individually (Fig 6).

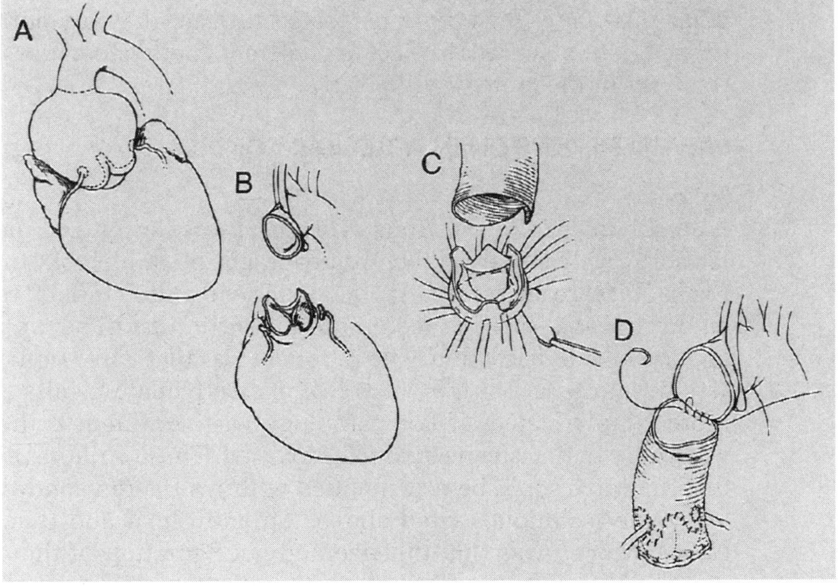

FIGURE 5.

Valve resuspension in a tubular conduit. **A,** the *dotted lines* indicate lines of resection. **B,** the aortic valve and coronary buttons are left intact. **C,** horizontal mattress sutures are placed subannularly. **D,** the valve is resuspended within the graft, and the distal end is anastomosed. (Adapted from David TE, Feindel CM: An aortic valve sparing operation for patients with aortic incompetence and aneurysm of the ascending aorta. *J Thorac Cardiovasc Surg* 103:617–622, 1992.)

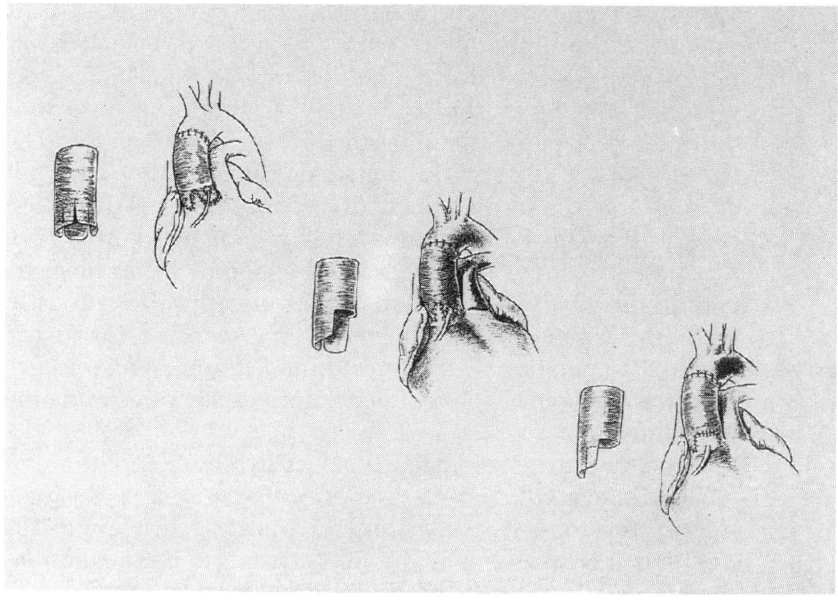

FIGURE 6.

Modifications of valve resuspension in a tubular conduit. The conduit is cut to replace one, two, or three individual sinuses. (Adapted from David TE, Feindel CM, Bos J: Repair of the aortic valve in patients with aortic insufficiency and aortic root aneurysm. *J Thorac Cardiovasc Surg* 109:345–352, 1995.)

Evaluation

This operation, as originally described, is theoretically very appealing, albeit somewhat technically formidable. It offers the possibility of a cure of the disease process by complete excision of the diseased aortic wall. Further, because the base of the graft is placed in a subvalvular or annular position, the technique offers long-term fixation of the aortic annulus. This point is important, because connective tissue diseases that involve the aortic root theoretically involve the endoskeleton of the heart. Therefore, a procedure such as this, which treats the aneurysmal disease from a subvalvular level up through the ascending aorta, cannot be criticized for leaving diseased tissue untreated. One major appeal of this procedure as originally described, therefore, is that recurrence of the disease is unlikely. This appeal is lost in the modified procedures that do not include subvalvular stitch placement.

The greatest theoretical drawback of the original procedure is that the durability of the "normal" aortic valve in an abnormal environment remains to be seen. David and Feindel[19] acknowledge that a straight tubular graft, without sinuses of Valsalva, may have detrimental effects during leaflet opening and may result in elevated stresses in the leaflets. In addition, because the native valve is to be spared, the relationship of the graft size and shape to the size of the leaflets may have significant effects on valve closure, leaflet stress, and longevity of the repair. It is therefore essential to understand the relationship between native aortic root size and shape and leaflet size and shape to accomplish this procedure effectively. Although this is a very appealing procedure, the technical demands, the required geometric understanding, and the necessary operative time have limited its use. For these reasons, surgeons have once again sought more expeditious and simplified procedures.

The modifications recently described by David et al.,[20] which exclude subvalvular stitch placement in favor of "tailoring" the sinuses, are more expedient but theoretically less appealing. This modification may benefit the operative time but abandons one of the original benefits of the procedure, i.e., fixation of the annulus. As the annulus is a subvalvular structure, it will not be subject to fixation by a supravalvular suture line.

CONDUIT REPLACEMENT WITH AORTIC ROOT INCLUSION

Rationale

Although similar to the procedure described by David, the technique described by Ergin and Griepp[21] is one attempt to simplify the approach and shorten operative time by reducing the number and complexity of the suture lines. This technique also uses a tubular conduit to remodel the aortic root wall.

Technique

In this procedure, the ascending aorta is transected approximately 15 mm above the plane of the aortic commissures. In contrast to the procedure described by David, the sinus tissue, including the coronary arteries, is left intact. The graft is therefore prepared with "keyholes" cut out to fit around the coronaries (Fig 7). A series of pledgeted sutures are placed to reshape the aortic valve and restore the competency of the valve. All these stitches, however, are placed in a supravalvular position at the top of the commissures and above the valve leaflets in the three sinuses. The graft is slipped over the proximal portion of the aorta, the pledgeted sutures are passed through the graft, and the keyholes are closed. The proximal cuff of the aortic root within the supporting graft is then circumferen-

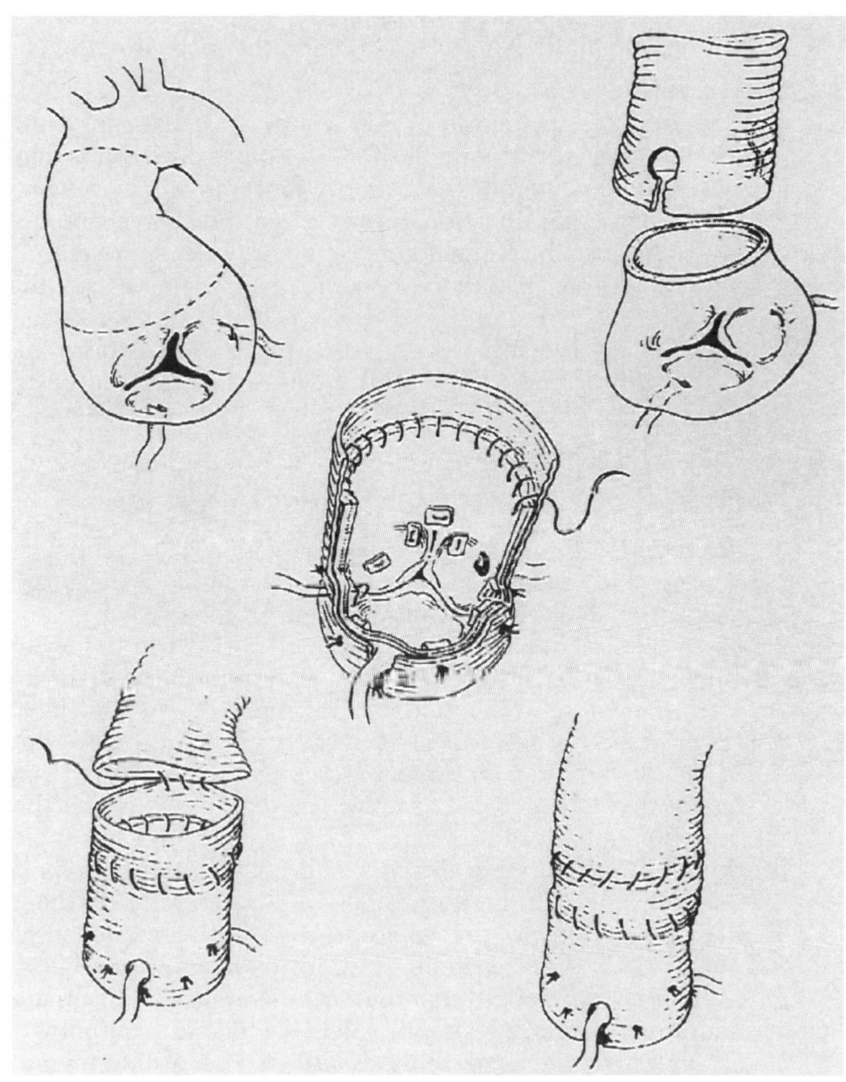

FIGURE 7.

Conduit replacement with aortic root inclusion. The entire aortic root is included (resuspended) within a conduit with keyholes cut out for the coronary arteries. (Courtesy of Ergin MA, Griepp RB: When, why and how should the native aortic valve be preserved in patients with anuloaortic ectasia or Marfan syndrome? *Semin Thorac Cardiovasc Surg* 5:93–96, 1993.)

tially sutured to the graft. The remainder of the ascending aortic aneurysm is replaced with a separate piece of graft, and a graft-to-graft anastomosis is used to complete the reconstruction.

Evaluation

The proposed advantage of this technique is that the suture lines for the valve are less complex than for other procedures that mimic freehand homograft reconstruction; thus, operative time may be reduced. This simplification, however, also creates several disadvantages. Because the annular stitches are actually supra-annular, they will not correct annular dilatation or prevent further dilatation. Also, in the setting of root dilatation, there is excess tissue in the sinuses and ascending aorta. Attempting to constrain this tissue within a prosthetic graft could create distortion and obstruction. Although this procedure does accomplish the goal of simplicity, it does not fully restore normal geometry.

CONDUIT TAILORING IN A SUPRAVALVULAR POSITION

Rationale

Sarsam and Yacoub[6] reported an alternative valve-sparing approach in 1993. This technique offers an innovative, anatomically based description of how to replace all aortic wall tissue above the valve. The aim of this procedure is to replace the diseased aortic wall tissue and, in the process, to reshape the anatomical annulus (as described in the paper) back to its normal geometry to restore valve competence and preserve the valve leaflets. The primary focus of this technique is to tailor the conduit to match the asymmetric details of the human aortic sinuses of Valsalva. However, the "annulus" cited in the title of this paper refers to the semilunar attachment of the leaflets (anatomical annulus), rather than to the ringlike junction of the aortic wall and ventricle (surgical annulus). This is an example of the difference in terminology sited in the introduction, in that the terms "surgical" and "anatomical" annulus are reversed. Despite the difference in terminology, this is an insightful and remarkably descriptive paper that reviews some fundamentals of aortic root anatomy.

Technique

The most appealing aspect of this procedure is that, similar to the one described by David, all possible aortic wall is excised and only the remnants necessary to preserve the coronary ostia and the valve leaflets are spared. The procedure differs from the original David procedure but is similar to David's own modifications in management of the conduit. The base of a prosthetic graft is incised longitudinally at three points that correspond to the anatomical location of the commissures, and the length of the incision is determined by the desired height of the commissural post (Fig 8). The graft is then cut into a crown shape, the commissural posts are fixed, the graft is attached to the aortic remnant above the valve leaflets, and the coronary buttons are anastomosed.

Evaluation

There are several appealing aspects of this technique. First, the unique crown-shaped incisions may allow for anatomical varia-

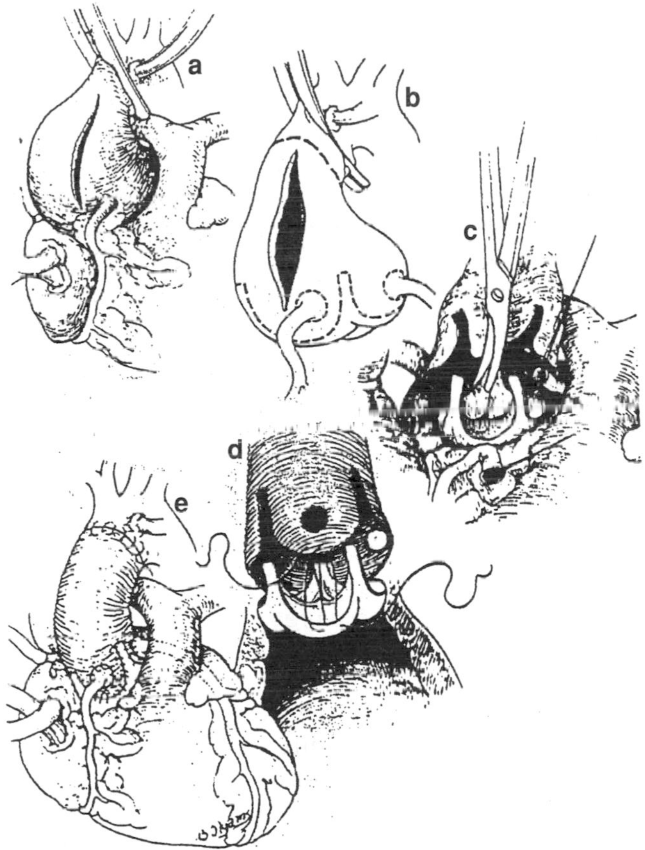

FIGURE 8.

Conduit tailoring in a supravalvular position. The graft is prepared in a crown shape, tailored to individual sinuses of Valsalva anatomy, and sutured to the aorta with reimplantation of coronary arteries. (Courtesy of Yacoub MH, Sundt TM, Rasmi N, et al: Management of aortic valve incompetence in patients with Marfan syndrome, in Hetzer R, Gehle P, Ennker J (eds.): *Cardiovascular Aspects of Marfan Syndrome.* New York, Springer Verlag, 1995, p 75.)

tions of the sinus of Valsalva regions in individual patients. Second, the shape may theoretically allow "bulging" of the graft that may simulate the shape of the natural sinuses. As such, this technique may be particularly applicable to such conditions as "isolated" aneurysm of the sinuses of Valsalva. The greatest appeal of this procedure, however, is that only one suture line is necessary at the valvular level; accordingly, the operative time may be decreased compared with other procedures.

There are, however, several drawbacks to this technique as well. The limitations are similar to those in the modified David procedures and the procedure described by Ergin and Griepp. With this technique, the aortic root pathology is assumed to be restricted to the aortic tissue in the sinuses, and the endoskeleton of the heart is not addressed. We do not support this premise in aortic root disease. If the disease is also present at the level of the subvalvular annulus, this technique will not suffice to remodel aortic tissue at that level because it is a supravalvular procedure, and subsequent dilatation is possible. This technique, therefore, is not as globally applicable to aortic root disease as the one that encompasses and constrains or "fixes" both the anatomical and surgical annulus.

CONDUIT TAILORING WITH PSEUDOSINUS CREATION

Rationale

As described previously, the aortic root is a complex system that relies on a balanced interaction of all components to attain efficient and durable function. The sinuses of Valsalva are crucial components for normal function of the aortic valve and root. As such, valve-sparing techniques must consider the role of the sinuses of Valsalva and, if possible, try to recreate them. The sinuses, in concert with the sinotubular junction, create eddy currents behind the valve leaflets, which initiate valve closure and promote coronary blood flow. This eddy formation assists in leaflet coaptation by ensuring early and coordinated closure of all three aortic leaflets. In addition, the curvilinear configuration created by the unique attachment of the aortic leaflets to the sinuses of Valsalva allows for stress sharing between the valve leaflets and aortic wall. Any aortic reconstruction that ignores and disrupts this complex stress-sharing configuration will result in increased leaflet stress, increased fatigue, and decreased durability of the valve.

In designing a procedure that treats aortic wall disease and offers the best chance of long-term durability, four principles for recreation of the complex aortic root interaction must be kept in mind. First, the aortic valve, once accessed and deemed salvageable, is spared and resuspended in as near normal environment as possible. Second, all abnormal tissue that can be excised is excised. Third, any remaining abnormal annular or valvular tissue must be secured to prosthetic material to prevent future dilation. Finally and most important, the sinuses of Valsalva and the sinotubular junction must be re-established. This last aspect is the most crucial, because it ensures that valve closure with its stress is accomplished and that coronary perfusion is maintained as close to normal as possible. An additional aspect of re-establishment of the sinuses configuration is the curvilinear orientation between leaflet and conduit wall, which is also stress reducing. To accomplish these goals, we have coupled concepts from the previously described surgical techniques with a means of recreating the sinuses of Valsalva.[22] The surgically created pseudosinus shape approximates the natural configuration. These pseudosinuses are designed to simulate and recreate the natural protective stress-sharing patterns that promote long-term durability of the native valve.

Creation of the pseudosinuses was theoretically based on increasing the proximal circumference of the conduit and then reducing its new increased length by fixation to the annulus, which, if appropriately sized, would be smaller. Fixation of the proximal end of the conduit and the commissural post results in bulging of the excess length of the conduit because of the increased circumference. The result is creation of pseudosinuses. In addition to appropriate formation and orientation of pseudosinuses, the commissural post fixation ensures re-creation of a sinotubular junction.

Before this technique was applied clinically, mathematical support for this concept was derived. Figure 9 illustrates the appearance of the modified free edge of the conduit, as if the conduit had been cut along its long axis and laid out flat. C_1 indicates the circumference of the unmodified conduit, and C_2 is the new free edge length of the modified conduit. If the scallops are considered symmetrical, the relationship between C_1 and C_2 can be based on the height (H) of the scallops that are cut into the graft. For the purpose of mathematical analysis, it is assumed that both the upper and lower curvatures of the scallop are arcs of a circle. The length of each of these arcs (three upper and three lower arcs) can be determined simply on the basis of the known diameter of the graft (D), and the chosen scallop height (H).

For each upper and lower scallop, the arc length(s) is defined by the formula

$s = R\theta$ where R = radius of circular arc (mm) and
θ is the angle (radians) (Equation 1).

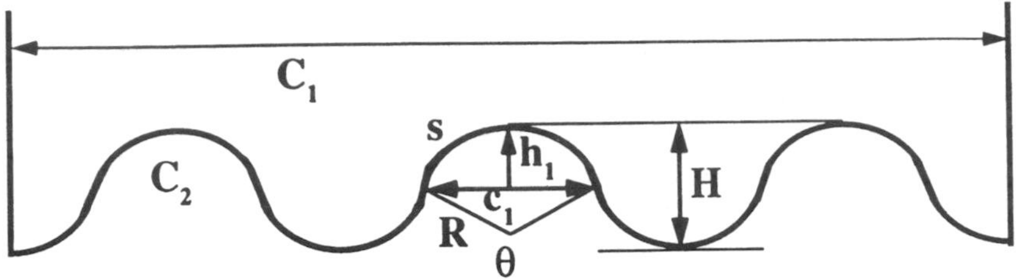

FIGURE 9.
Measurements used for mathematical derivation of increased length from C_1 (original circumference of conduit) to C_2 (modified circumference of conduit). (Courtesy of Cochran RP, Kunzelman KS, Eddy AC, et al: Modified conduit preparation creates a pseudosinus in an aortic valve sparing procedure for aneurysm of the ascending aorta. *J Thorac Cardiovasc Surg* 109:1049–1058, 1995.)

Although R and θ are not directly known, they can be calculated from the chord length c_1 and arc height h_1. The trigonometric formula that defines the relationship is

$$c_1 = \sqrt{4h_1(2R-h_1)} \qquad \text{(Equation 2).}$$

Solving for R gives

$$R = \frac{c_1^{\,2} + 4h_1^{\,2}}{8h_1} \qquad \text{(Equation 3).}$$

Next, the trigonometric formula defining the angle θ is

$$\theta = 2\sin^{-1}\frac{c_1}{2R} \qquad \text{(Equation 4).}$$

Substituting Equation 3 into 4 gives

$$\theta = 2\sin^{-1}\frac{4h_1c_1}{c_1^{\,2} + 4h_1^{\,2}} \qquad \text{(Equation 5).}$$

Substituting Equations 3 and 5 for Equation 1 gives the arc length based only on chord length and height:

$$s = \frac{c_1^{\,2} + 4h_1^{\,2}}{4h_1}\sin^{-1}\frac{4h_1c_1}{c_1^{\,2} + 4h_1^{\,2}} \qquad \text{(Equation 6).}$$

Finally, knowing that c_1 is equivalent to one sixth the original circumference (C_1, which can be calculated from the diameter) and that h_1 is one half the scallop height (H), the final equation for the new free edge length (C_2) of the modified conduit is six times the arc length *s*, or

$$C_2 = 6s = \frac{(\pi D)^2 + 36H^2}{12H} \sin^{-1} \frac{12\pi DH}{(\pi D)^2 + 36H^2}$$
(Equation 7).

The relationship between scallop height and resultant modified free edge length is shown for varying graft diameters in Figure 10. As illustrated, a significant increase in free edge length can be achieved by scalloping the graft. Figure 11 shows the idealized geometric result. A crucial aspect of this reconstruction is that the new free edge length (C_2) is attached to the subvalvular annular circumference (C_1) in the same horizontal plane of the surgical annulus, not the crown-shaped anatomical annulus. Fixation of the conduit at this level ensures fixation of the endoskeleton of the heart and should prevent long-term dilation and preserve the newly reconstructed aortic root. The reconstruction of the conduit into an aortic root is completed by symmetrical fixation of the three commissural posts. The physical result is that the extra material "created" by the scallops will be forced to bulge upward and outward, thereby creating pseudosinuses.

In addition to creating pseudosinuses, we wanted to know the amount of bulging that could be created, so the maximum degree

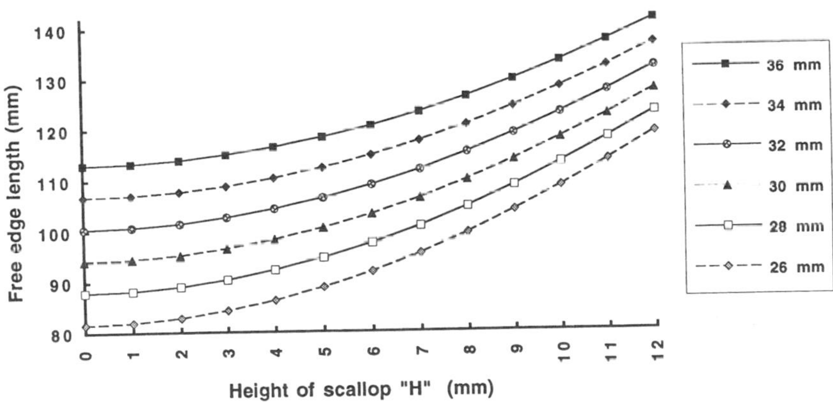

FIGURE 10.
Graphic representation of increase in free edge length (modified circumference for various scallop heights (*H*) for several conduit sizes. (Courtesy of Cochran RP, Kunzelman KS, Eddy AC, et al: Modified conduit preparation creates a pseudosinus in an aortic valve sparing procedure for aneurysm of the ascending aorta. *J Thorac Cardiovasc Surg* 109:1049–1058, 1995.)

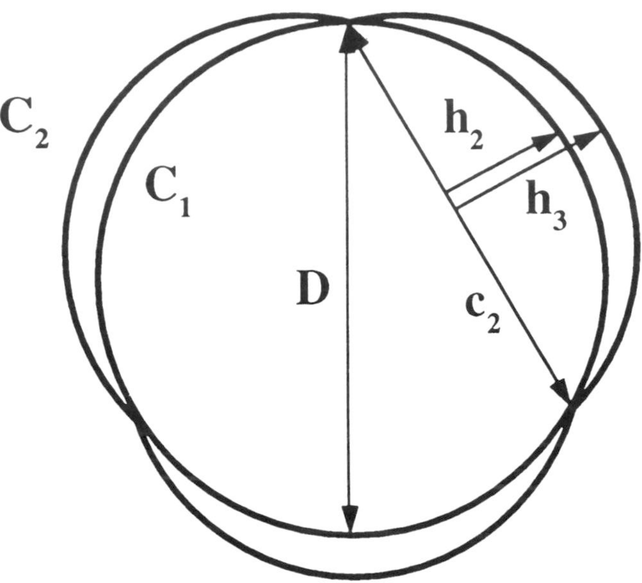

FIGURE 11.
Idealized geometric configuration attained with new free edge length (C_2) attached to annular circumference (C_1) and commissural posts and the additional sinus depth that results (h_3–h_2). (Courtesy of Cochran RP, Kunselman KS, Eddy AC, et al: Modified conduit preparation creates a pseudosinus in an aortic valve sparing procedure for aneurysm of the ascending aorta. *J Thorac Cardiovasc Surg* 109:1049–1058, 1995.)

of bulging, or "additional sinus depth," was also calculated by trigonometric relationships. The numerical value of the additional sinus depth is $h_3 - h_2$. Once again, assuming circular arcs, the relationship among chord length (c), chord height (h), and arc length (s), defined in Equation 6, holds true. In this case, the chord length c_2 is constant (and can be calculated from diameter, D). The two arc lengths of interest are equivalent to one third of C_1 and C_2 respectively. The values for h_2 and h_3 can then be solved implicitly from Equation 6. The relationship between scallop height and resultant additional sinus depth is shown for varying graft diameters in Figure 12. It can be seen that a definable increase in sinus depth can be gained by scalloping the graft.

Technique

For the modified technique, the conduit was trimmed to create three symmetrical scallops in the annular end of the Dacron conduit; each scallop had a maximal height of 5–7 mm, depending on conduit size. Other than the difference in trimming of the base of the conduit, the technique of insertion is similar to that described by David. One important difference, however, is subvalvular suture placement. To attain fixation of the endoskeleton of the heart, the horizontal mattress stitches are placed in the plane of the subvalvular annulus and do not follow the curve of the surgical or crown-shaped annulus in any of the commissural regions. Other than this significant difference in fixation of the annulus, the technique is very similar and includes placement of the subvalvular stitches along the proximal end of the conduit, resuspension of the valve within the conduit, and reimplantation of the coronary arteries (Fig 13).

Evaluation

The creation of pseudosinuses was confirmed intraoperatively by visual inspection and postoperatively by echocardiography. Figures 14 A and B show echocardiogram images (short and long axis views) from the first patient in whom we undertook valve sparing for aortic aneurysmal disease with the technique originally described by David. On echocardiogram, there is no evidence of sinus formation. In contrast, Figures 14 C and D show echocardiogram images (short and long axis view) of a patient in whom we

Additional sinus depth calculated from scallop height

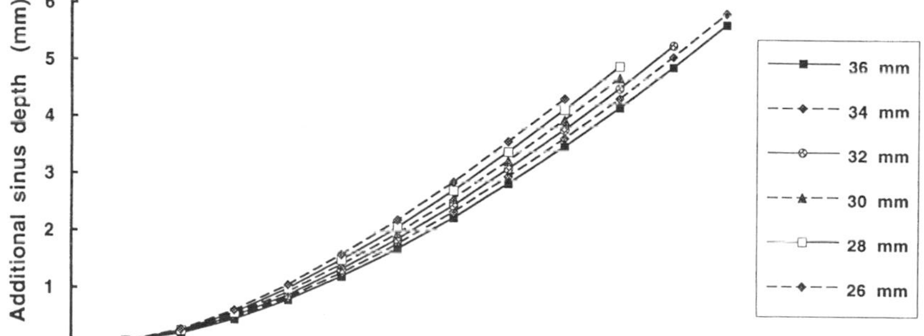

FIGURE 12.

Graphic representation of the relationship between scallop height and the resultant additional sinus depth shown for several conduit sizes. (Courtesy of Cochran RP, Kunzelman KS, Eddy AC, et al: Modified conduit preparation creates a pseudosinus in an aortic valve sparing procedure for aneurysm of the ascending aorta. *J Thorac Cardiovasc Surg* 109:1049–1058, 1995.)

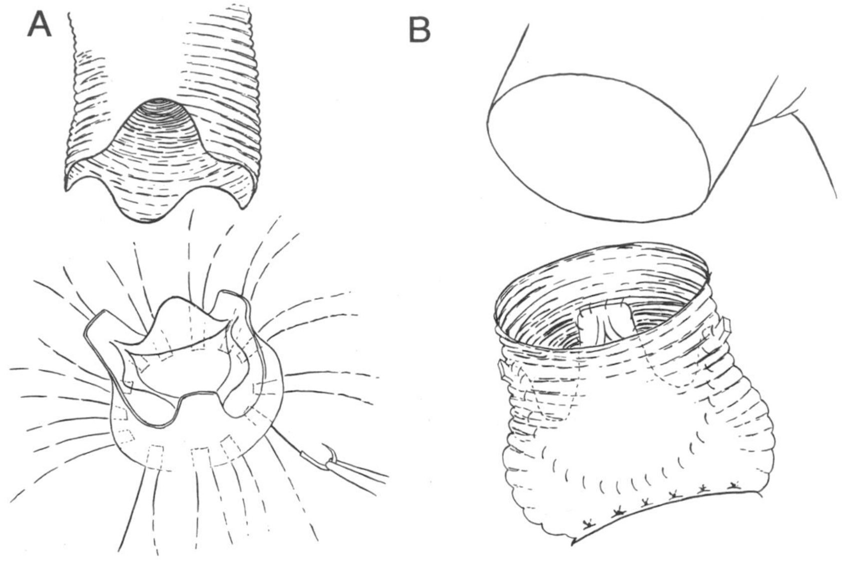

FIGURE 13.

A, creation of three symmetrical scallops in the proximal conduit and circumferential subvalvular stitch placement. **B,** Completed conduit placement and valve resuspension with creation of "pseudo-sinuses." (Courtesy of Cochran RP, Kunzelman KS, Eddy AC, et al: Modified conduit preparation creates a pseudosinus in an aortic valve sparing procedure for aneurysm of the ascending aorta. *J Thorac Cardiovasc Surg* 109:1049–1058, 1995.)

used the modified pseudosinus technique. The constructed pseudosinuses are apparent in both views. In addition, in the long axis view, the leaflets appear to retract naturally without contact to the conduit walls.

We believe that this pseudosinus procedure is superior to the other valve-sparing procedures because it adheres to the four goals established for best results in recreation of the aortic root: It allows for sparing of any salvageable valves. It removes the maximal amount of diseased tissue. It "fixes" all remaining tissue so that further dilatation cannot occur. Finally, and most significantly, it returns the spared aortic valve to a more natural environment that allows for the natural stress-sharing mechanisms of the aortic root to be recreated. This procedure, however, shares one potential drawback with all other techniques. All the aortic valve–sparing reconstructions currently use a synthetic conduit. Unfortunately, all available synthetic conduits have mechanical properties that are

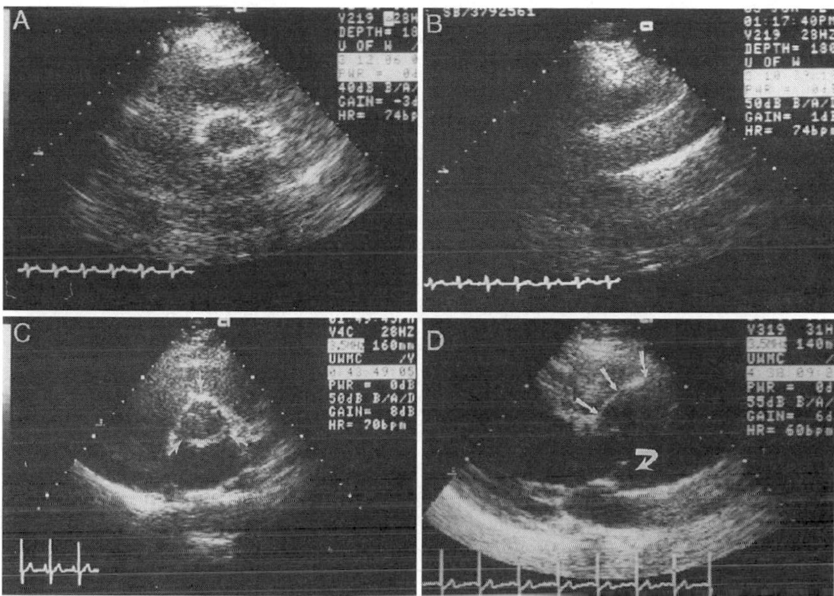

FIGURE 14.

Short axis **(A)** and long axis **(B)** echocardiogram from first patient (without modified conduit) demonstrates no sinus formation. **C,** short axis view from patient with modified conduit demonstrates pseudosinuses, depicted by the *three arrows.* **D,** Long axis view of patient with modified conduit demonstrates curvilinear attachment of conduit to annulus, pseudosinus formation marked by *three arrows* and the aortic leaflet retracting into a "sinus" space shown by the *curved arrow.* (Courtesy of Cochran RP, Kunzelman KS, Eddy AC, et al: Modified conduit preparation creates a pseudosinus in an aortic valve sparing procedure for aneurysm of the ascending aorta. *J Thorac Cardiovasc Surg* 109:1049–1058, 1995.)

significantly different from the native aorta. The available synthetic conduits are much less compliant and, therefore, do not expand as the native aorta would. This difference in compliance may, in and of itself, change the stress patterns in the valve. Because of the unknown effect of the difference in mechanical properties of synthetic conduits vs. aorta, the long-term durability of these techniques is yet to be determined.

CANDIDATES FOR AORTIC VALVE SPARING

Valve-sparing operations are best suited for patients whose aortic valves have a good potential of being returned to normal (or near normal) function. For example, patients who have clearly isolated acute aortic wall disease, such as an acute dissection, are ideal. In addition, patients who have aneurysmal disease, but with an aortic valve that is structurally intact and undamaged, are also appropriate for valve-sparing procedures. It is in this group of patients, in particular, that we advocate early treatment, rather than the "watchful waiting" that has been historically associated with the timing of intervention for aortic aneurysms. The longer the aneurysm is present, the longer the period of abnormal stress, which may subsequently damage the leaflets and negate the opportunity for valve sparing.

In contrast to patients who have dissection or aneurysm but relatively normal valves, patients who have stenotic valvular lesions that require significant leaflet tissue mobilization or replacement remain poor candidates for valve-sparing operations. The literature to date supports this statement, in that the reported attempts at sparing the stenotic aortic valve have not shown good results, even in the short term. An additional concern regarding the present state of valve sparing for stenosis is that the nature of the reparative techniques has varied, and the indications have not been made clear in the published reports. At present, we cannot advocate sparing the valve in these patients.

Despite this fairly rigorous patient restriction, the number of patients who are anatomically and physiologically suited for aortic valve–sparing operations is increasing. From 1965 to 1975, the prevalence of annular dilation in patients who underwent surgery for pure aortic insufficiency was 17%.[23] In 1980, the reported incidence of annular dilatation increased to 37%.[24] In 1990, it had increased to 50%,[25] thereby making annular dilatation the single most common cause of aortic insufficiency in North America. As such, there is and will be a greater demand for cardiac surgery that is appropriate for these patients.

In patients who have aortic root dilatation, two principal groups, based on age, emerge. The first group consists of patients who are in the first six decades of life and who usually have Marfan's syndrome or another connective tissue abnormality. The second group consist of patients in the last three decades of life who have age-related degenerative problems. Valve-sparing procedures are very appealing to both groups but for different reasons. The younger patients generally have a strong desire to maintain an active lifestyle and have a greater life expectancy; as such, they usually prefer to avoid the anticoagulation required with mechanical valves. Younger patients also want to avoid the obligatory reoperation necessitated in most biological valve options. For these patients, a valve-sparing procedure offers an attractive alternative.

In the older age group, valve-sparing procedures are popular for the avoidance of anticoagulation and its complications, particularly those that increase as the patients enter the eighth and ninth decades of life. Both patient groups are increasing in size because of earlier diagnosis of the connective tissue diseases and the increasing age of the population. As a result, both groups are increasingly referred for surgical consideration for aortic insufficiency and aortic root dilatation, and more of the patients who are referred are interested in aortic valve–sparing operations.

Unfortunately, not all patients referred for aortic valve–sparing operations are good candidates for this type of procedure. Ultimately, the appropriateness of an aortic valve–sparing operation is limited by the state of the aortic leaflet tissue, i.e., there must be normal or near normal tissue present. This limitation is similar to those now encountered with mitral valve repair. Hopefully, with an increased understanding of disease processes, aortic valve and root system biomechanics, and customized materials design, the indications for procedures to spare the aortic valve will be extended to include many more patients. At present, several potential techniques have been described for patients who are currently selected for the procedure. We believe strongly that the best long-term results will be attained by recreating an environment as near to normal as possible for the "spared" aortic valve. We therefore believe that the procedure of choice is aortic valve sparing coupled with creation of pseudosinuses. The procedure, as we have designed it, is simple and reproducible and has had gratifying results with both short and intermediate follow-up.

CONCLUSION

The sparing of the aortic valve in selected cases of aortic insufficiency is an excellent alternative to procedures that require mechanical valve replacement. The ideal procedure and the ideal materials for reconstruction of the aortic root continue to evolve. As the incidence of aortic root abnormalities increases, cardiac surgeons must become facile in the management of this previously formidable region. If current trends continue, the next decade promises to increase the need for this type of surgical option significantly. Unfortunately, the long-term durability of the aortic valve in an artificial conduit will remain questionable until long-term follow-up is complete. It seems intuitive that as valve-sparing procedures more closely approximate the natural anatomical arrangement, that resultant biomechanics and long-term durability will be improved. As described, the introduction of a simple scalloped modification of the prosthetic graft end allows for creation of pseudosinuses adjacent to the valve leaflets. For patients who have aortic root aneurysms and dissections, with normal or near normal aortic valves, this modified aortic valve–sparing, aortic root replacement is the procedure of choice.

REFERENCES

1. Robiscek F: Leonardo da Vinci and the sinuses of Valsalva. *Ann Thorac Surg* 52:328–335, 1991.
2. *Stedman's Dictionary,* ed 22. Baltimore, Md, Williams and Wilkins, 1972.
3. *Dorland's Illustrated Medical Dictionary,* ed 24. Philadelphia, WB Saunders, 1965.
4. Gray H: *Gray's Anatomy.* Philadelphia, Lea and Febiger, 1973.
5. Anderson JE: *Grant's Atlas of Anatomy,* ed 8. Balitmore, Md, Williams & Wilkins.
6. Sarsam MAI, Yacoub M: Remodeling of the aortic valve anulus. *J Thorac Cardiovasc Surg* 105:435–438, 1993.
7. Bentall H, DeBono A: A technique for complete replacement of the ascending aorta. *Thorax* 23:338–339, 1968.
8. Angell WW, Oury JH, Shah P: A comparison of replacement and reconstruction in patients with mitral regurgitation. *J Thorac Cardiovasc Surg* 93:665–674, 1987.
9. Perier P, Deloche A. Comparative evaluation of mitral valve repair and replacement with Starr, Bjork, and porcine valve prostheses. *Circulation* 70:I-187–I-192, 1984.
10. Bernal JM, Rabasa JM, Cagigas JC, et al: Valve-related complications with the Hancock I porcine bioprosthesis: A twelve to fourteen year follow-up study. *J Thorac Cardiovasc Surg* 101:871–880, 1991.
11. Antunes MJ: Techniques of valvular reoperation. *Eur J Cardiothor Surg* 6:54S–58S, 1992.
12. Groves LK, Effler DB, Hank WA, et al: Aortic insufficiency secondary to aneurysmal changes in the ascending aorta: Surgical management. *J Thorac Cardiovasc Surg* 48:362–379, 1964.
13. Kouchoukos NT, Karp RB, Blackstone EH, et al: Replacement of the ascending aorta and aortic valve with a composite graft. *Ann Surg* 192:403–413, 1980.
14. Massimo CG, Presenti LF, Marronci P, et al: Extended and total aortic resection in the surgical treatment of acute type A aortic dissection. *Ann Thorac Surg* 46:420–421, 1988.
15. DeBakey ME, McCollum CH, Crawford ES, et al: Dissection and dissecting aneurysms of the aorta: Twenty-year follow-up of five hundred twenty-seven patients treated surgically. *Surgery* 92:118–134, 1982.
16. Miller DC: Aortic dissection, aneurysm, and trauma and congenital disease of the aorta. *Curr Opin Cardiol* 4:693–704, 1989.

17. Miller DC, Stinson EB, Oyer PE, et al: Operative treatment of aortic dissections. *J Thorac Cardiovasc Surg* 78:365–382, 1979.
18. Najafi H, Dye WS, Javid H, et al: Acute aortic regurgitation secondary to aortic dissection. *Ann Thorac Surg* 14:474–482, 1972.
19. David TE, Feindel CM: An aortic valve sparing operation for patients with aortic incompetence and aneurysm of the ascending aorta. *J Thorac Cardiovasc Surg* 103:617–622, 1992.
20. David RE, Feindel CM, Bos J: Repair of the aortic valve in patients with aortic insufficiency and aortic root aneurysm. *J Thorac Cardiovasc Surg.* 109:345–352, 1995.
21. Ergin MA, Griepp RB: When, why, and how should the native aortic valve be preserved in patient with annuloaortic ectasia or Marfan syndrome. *Semin Thorac Cardiovasc Surg* 5:91–92, 1993.
22. Cochran RP, Kunzelman KS, Eddy AC, et al: Modified conduit preparation creates a pseudo-sinus in an aortic valve sparing procedure for ascending aortic aneurysm. *J Thor Cardiovasc Surg* 109:1049–1058, 1995.
23. Davies MH: *Pathology of Cardiac Valves.* Toronto, Butterworths, 1980, pp 37–61.
24. Olson LJ, Subramanian R, Edwards WD: Surgical pathology of pure aortic insufficiency: A study of 225 cases. *Mayo Clin Proc* 59:835–841, 1984.
25. Dare AH, Veinot JP, Edwards WE, et al: New observations on the etiology of aortic valve disease: A surgical pathologic study of 236 cases from 1990. *Hum Pathol* 24:1330–1338, 1993.

Conduits in the Pulmonary Circulation

John W. Brown, M.D.
Harris B. Shumaker Professor of Surgery and Chief, Section of Cardiovascular Surgery, Indiana University School of Medicine, Indianapolis

Thomas X. Aufiero, M.D.
Associate Professor of Surgery, Indiana University School of Medicine, Indianapolis

Kung Sun, M.D., Ph.D.
Korea University Medical Center, Seoul

Extracardiac conduits between the right ventricle (RV) and the pulmonary artery (PA) have allowed the repair of multiple congenital malformations, including truncus arteriosus, pulmonary atresia with a ventricular septal defect (PA/VSD), transposition of the great vessels (TGV), tetralogy of Fallot (TOF), and other complex entities. Over the years, many different conduit types have been proposed. Klinner and Zenker,[1] and Rastelli et al.[2] reported the use of nonvalved conduits in 1965. Ross and Somerville[3] reported the first use of a homograft conduit for the correction of pulmonary atresia in 1966, and Bowman et al.[4] reported the use of porcine valved Dacron conduits in 1973. Despite excellent early results after conduit reconstruction of the right ventricular outflow tract (RVOT), these extracardiac conduits still represent one of the ongoing weak links in reconstructive congenital heart surgery. Conduit failures from neointimal ingrowth, thrombus formation, and valve deterioration in Dacron and xenograft conduits and from stenosis and calcification in homograft conduits continue to limit the durability of these repairs and commit most patients to multiple operations. An emphasis on earlier repair in younger infants has amplified some of these conditions and has added the additional problem of patients who may outgrow their conduit.

An increasing interest in pulmonary autograft replacement of the aortic valve (the Ross procedure) for younger patients who have aortic valve problems will create another group of patients with homograft RVOT reconstruction. Although the early and midterm

© 1996, Mosby–Year Book, Inc.

results of homograft function in this setting have been quite good, questions regarding the long-term function of the homograft and possible failure mechanisms remain. Investigations into the immunologic behavior of homografts continue in the hope of reducing, or eliminating, some types of failure. In addition, the availability and difficulty in procuring homograft valves leads us to continue the evaluation of other materials and methods for RVOT reconstruction.

TECHNIQUE OF RIGHT VENTRICLE TO PULMONARY ARTERY CONDUIT PLACEMENT

ALLOGRAFT VALVE COLLECTION TECHNIQUES

Both aortic and pulmonary valve allografts, along with the respective ascending and transverse aorta or the PA and right and left branch PAs, are obtained either at the time of multiple organ retrieval or at the time of autopsy. It is important that the donor be screened and has met all the age and health criteria. Through a median sternotomy, the heart, ascending aorta, and PAs are removed in the same manner as for cardiac transplantation. The heart is immersed in saline to remove gross blood clot from the ventricular chambers and the great vessels. The heart can then be placed in a sterile container and Hanks' balanced salt solution at 4° centigrade for transportation. In the United States, most valves are now prepared by commercial organizations. If necessary, however, the dissection can be done by the surgeon. The epicardium is raised and dissected from the aorta down to the aortic root. The coronary arteries are identified, ligated with ties of heavy silk, and divided 3–4 mm from the ostia. The aorta is then separated from the PA. When the septal myocardium is located, it is incised with great care not to cut through the membranous septum. The dissection is then carried toward the left atrium, and the mitral valve is exposed. The mitral valve is dissected and remains with the aortic allograft. Excess myocardium is trimmed away from the aortic root. Gentle placement of a finger through the valve from below helps in this maneuver. A remnant of approximately 5–6 mm of myocardium should remain on the allograft. The valve cusps are then carefully inspected. Small fenestrations are acceptable. The pulmonary valve is then removed in a similar fashion (Fig 1). The valves can be sized by passing Hagar dilators into the annulus. Cultures of all valves are obtained, and the valves are routinely stored in liquid nitrogen. When needed, the allograft is removed from its container and is placed in a saline solution at 42° centigrade. With the use of a sterile technique, the allograft is then removed from its container

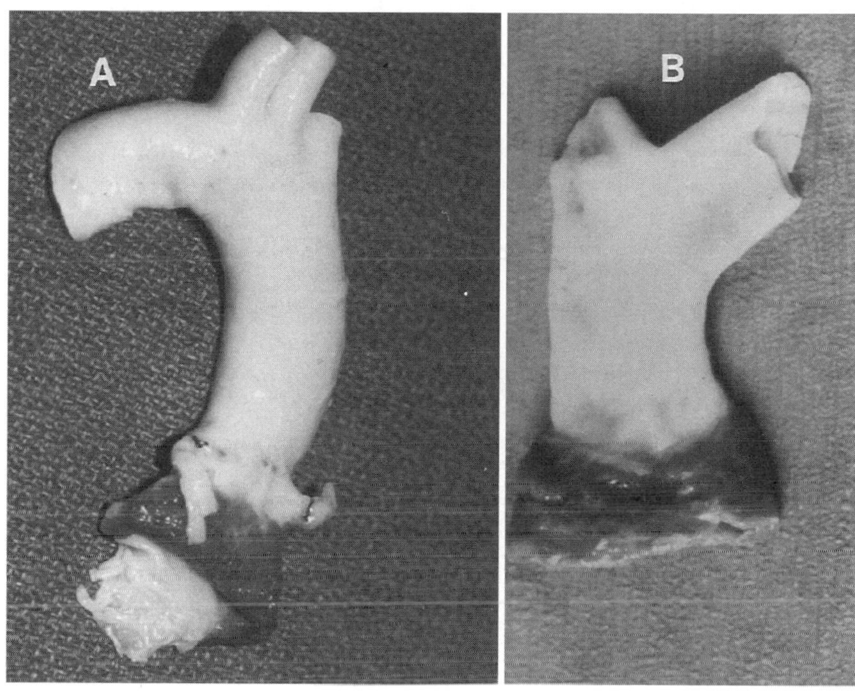

FIGURE 1.
A, aortic homograft after excision. Note the ligated coronary arteries and the attached anterior mitral leaflet. **B,** pulmonary homograft after excision. Note the cuff of right ventricular muscle and the stumps of the proximal branch pulmonary arteries.

and placed in tissue culture fluid with 10% dimethylsulfoxide at 42° centigrade. The valve is then washed in three separate rinses of tissue culture fluid. It is now ready for trimming and use as replacement.[5]

TECHNIQUE OF PRIMARY RIGHT VENTRICLE TO PULMONARY ARTERY CONDUIT CONSTRUCTION

A median sternotomy is performed in the standard fashion. Cannulation for cardiopulmonary bypass is modified depending on the underlying congenital lesion and the size of the patient. We favor the use of two venous cannulas in most instances, but a single venous cannula works well for neonates. Deep hypothermia and circulatory arrest is not used even in the smallest infants. Multiple dose crystalloid cardioplegia (15 mL/kg/dose) is used in infants who weigh less than 10 kg, whereas larger patients receive multiple-dose blood cardioplegia. Retrograde coronary sinus car-

Evaluation

These early techniques of valve resuspension had two very appealing aspects. First, all the techniques spared the aortic valve and, as such, hopefully avoided valve-related complications. Second, and more compelling, as facility was gained with valve resuspension, these techniques actually shortened the operative intervention in a complex, high-risk patient population.

Unfortunately, there are potential drawbacks with these techniques. Valve resuspension in the dissected aorta does not remove all abnormal tissue, particularly in the sinuses of Valsalva. This remaining tissue represents a continued risk for further dissection or aneurysm formation. One further limitation to widespread acceptance of this procedure was that in the era that this technique was first described, the procedure was not applied to aneurysmal disease in the ascending aorta. Instead, the technique used for aneurysmal disease was either composite valve-conduit replacement or supracoronary graft replacement with or without valve replacement. The latter technique neglected the fact that any aortic wall tissue left in place was subject to recurrent aneurysmal disease, particularly in the sinuses of Valsalva.

VALVE RESUSPENSION IN A TUBULAR CONDUIT

Rationale

As techniques for dissections evolved, it was recognized that similar aortic valve–sparing techniques might be applicable for aneurysmal disease as well. In April 1992, David and Feindel[19] reported an aortic valve–sparing technique for aortic insufficiency in both aneurysm and dissection. The rationale was that valve replacement was not necessary if the valve leaflets were anatomically normal. More simply stated, if the pathology was confined to the aortic wall, only that tissue needed to be excised. These authors proposed that the valve could be resuspended within a Dacron conduit, similar to the techniques cited above. An additional and crucial feature, however, was that the size and configuration of the conduit were used to restore a normal annular diameter. This aspect of annular fixation is one of the critical aspects in treating the diseased aortic root and attaining durable long-term results.

Technique

In this technique, the ascending aorta is transected just beyond the aneurysmal dilatation, and all three sinuses of Valsalva are excised, leaving 5–7 mm of arterial wall attached to the aortic valve and a dioplegia is used when there is associated aortic valve regurgitation. The PA is usually incised to the left of the aortic arch. The ventricle is then opened in a longitudinal fashion at its highest point. Care is taken to avoid major coronary branches and the aortic valve in TGV. The ventriculotomy should not be closer than 5 mm to any major coronary vessels. A VSD can often be closed through this incision. Alternatively, it can be closed through the right atrium. Regardless of whether a porcine valved Dacron conduit or a valved homograft conduit is used, the distal anastomosis is constructed first. The valve is placed as close to the PA as possible. The use of a pulmonary homograft allows extension onto the distal PAs to enlarge a stenosis. The use of the entire bifurcation and branch PAs allows the reconstruction of an atretic PA. The ventriculotomy can be undercut as necessary to allow for unobstructed egress from the RV cavity. The distal anastomosis is usually constructed with a continuous 5-0 polypropylene suture in older patients; in neonates, however, a 5-0 or 6-0 absorbable monofilament suture is used. If a Dacron valved conduit is used, the proximal end is tailored to fit the ventriculotomy and is sutured in place with a continuous 4-0 polypropylene suture. When a homograft valve is used, the allograft is extended proximally with an expanded polytetrafluoroethylene (PTFE) ringed graft to facilitate attachment to the RVOT. The ringed PTFE graft helps maintain the circular orifice of the homograft annulus. The valve itself is positioned perpendicular to the RV free wall. The proximal end of the PTFE hood is tapered to facilitate attachment to the right ventriculotomy (Fig 2). In some institutions, Dacron has been used for this proximal patch and also to extend some of the shorter pulmonary allografts. We try to avoid this approach if at all possible, as the neointimal buildup in Dacron may severely limit the life span of the graft.

As large a conduit as can safely be accommodated in the mediastinum should be used. This approach allows for continued growth without causing a functional stenosis. In addition, larger conduits seem to perform better than smaller conduits. However, the conduit must not be so large as to angulate at the distal anastomosis, which could cause distortion of the PAs, compression of the coronary artery, or compression of the conduit between the sternum and the heart. In the past when an aortic homograft was used, it was placed with the convex curve away from the aorta. This approach positions the conduit lateral to the sternum and decreases the possibilities of compression. In our current practice, aortic homografts are only used for RV to PA reconstruction in situations where the pulmonary vascular resistance is significantly elevated.

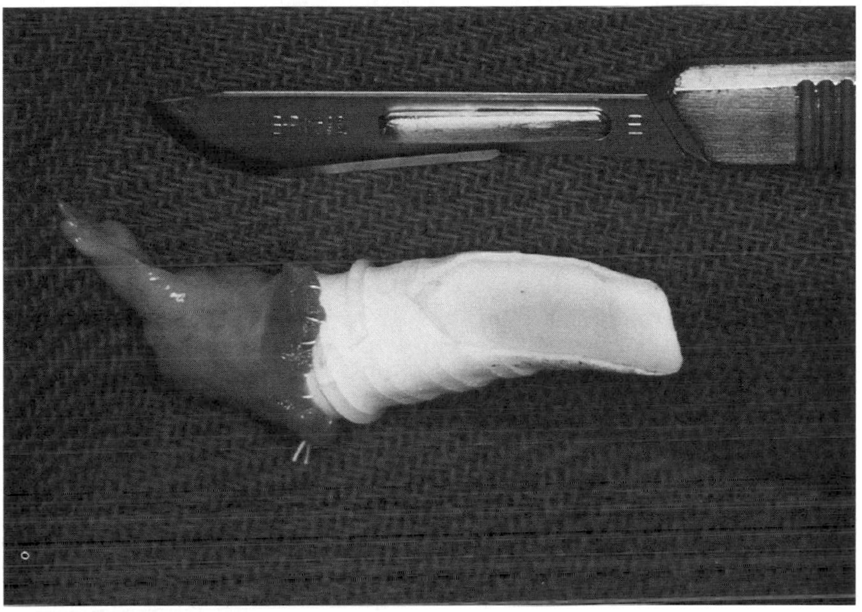

FIGURE 2.
Pulmonary homograft conduit with proximal extension using a ringed expanded polytetrafluoroethylene graft.

CONDUIT REPLACEMENT

Sternal re-entry, in patients who have had previous RV to PA conduits can be hazardous if the conduit is close or adherent to the posterior table of the sternum. This situation is more common with a Dacron valved conduit replacement than with a homograft replacement. We routinely prepare and drape the groins so that femoral-femoral bypass can be instituted if necessary. In patients about whom there is great concern regarding adherence to the posterior table of the sternum, a preoperative CT scan can further evaluate this situation. If the sternum appears to be adherent to the graft, femoral-femoral bypass can be instituted before dividing the posterior table of the sternum. Because of the need for frequent reentry for conduit change and the concerns of conduit adherence to the sternum, we routinely close the pericardium with a 0.1-mm expanded PTFE patch.

In most cases, if no other intracardiac corrections are necessary, the conduit replacement can be performed on a beating heart. We often use a single-stage venous cannula placed in the right atrium. The conduit is then identified and dissected anteriorly. It is opened on its anterior surface, and any thrombus present is removed. The proximal attachment is then removed, which leaves a firm fibrous rim on the ventricular side for suturing the new conduit in place. Dacron conduits are encapsulated in a dense fibrous tissue and can usually be peeled out. Distally, the conduit is excised at the PA anastomosis, which leaves fresh PA. If there is narrowing of the branch PAs, the incision is extended through the stenotic area. Pulmonary arteries can be augmented with a patch of autologous pericardium, xeno pericardium, or expanded PTFE. If a homograft is used, homograft tissue can be used to augment the PA as needed. Again, the distal anastomosis is constructed first. The remainder of the procedure is performed as described previously for the primary operation.

In our current practice, we rarely use a second valved conduit (Dacron or homograft) in patients who require reoperation for RV to PA conduit dysfunction or outgrowth. Before June 1994, a homograft conduit that was not calcified was incised longitudinally and augmented with a simple expanded PTFE patch (0.4–0.6 mm thick) sewn to the edges of the split homograft. In instances where a densely calcified homograft (usually an aortic) is encountered, the homograft is split longitudinally and the calcium debrided, thereby leaving a fibrous posterior capsule. A simple patch is fashioned from 0.4 or 0.6–mm expanded PTFE to the posterior fibrous capsule to augment the RV to PA pathway.

In the replacement of a Dacron valved conduit, the conduit is split anteriorly, and all the Dacron is excised, thereby leaving a dense, nearly circumferential fibrous bed. This fibrous bed is then simply roofed with an expanded PTFE patch. Since June 1994, nearly all patients who have required conduit changes have been treated as outlined above, with the exception that a somewhat redundant 0.1–mm expanded PTFE monocusp is inserted under the PTFE RVOT pathway. This same technique is used primarily in all patients who have TOF and are undergoing transannular reconstruction of the RVOT. Results to date, although short-term, have been encouraging.

THE INDIANA UNIVERSITY EXPERIENCE WITH RIGHT VENTRICLE TO PULMONARY ARTERY CONDUITS

The experience with conduit reconstruction of the RVOT at Indiana University from February 1974 through August 1995 was reviewed. During this time, 159 conduits were implanted in 84 male and 56 female patients. The patients were aged 7 days to 50 years (mean age, 5.7 years) and weighed 2.5–105 kg (mean weight, 14.5 kg). Forty-four patients in this series had PA/VSD, and 40 had truncus arteriosus. Twenty-three patients had TGV, 13 had double outlet right ventricle (DORV), and 5 had complicated TOF. We have recently begun to use the Ross procedure with increasing frequency, and 15 patients in this series had reconstruction of the RVOT with a pulmonary homograft in association with this procedure. Seventy-five of the 140 patients (54%) had a second associated cardiac malformation, 16 of which involved an anomaly of the coronary arteries. Ninety-nine patients (71%) had undergone a previous operation before the definitive surgery involving the creation of the RV to PA conduit. Several patients had more than one procedure. Blalock-Taussig shunts were created in 97 patients, and Waterston-style shunts were created in 9. Pulmonary artery bands were placed in 5 patients, and 16 had a previous RVOT patch reconstruction. The interval between the palliative procedure and conduit placement ranged from 2 to 362 months (average interval, 67 months).

During the primary operation, a nonvalved conduit was placed in 41 patients, and a valved conduit was used in the reconstruction in 99 patients. These conduits ranged in size from 8 to 29 mm (mean size, 17 mm). The conduit size index (CSI) was determined according to the following formula: CSI = conduit size (mm)/patient weight (kilogram). In this series, the CSI ranged from 0.2 to 4.0 mm/kg (mean CSI, 1.2 mm/kg). Both xenograft and homograft valve conduits were used. Hancock valve conduits were used in 16 patients. Three patients each received a Bovine pericardial valve conduit or a mechanical valve conduit. Of the 77 homografts used for primary reconstruction, 49 were pulmonary homografts. These data are summarized in Table 1. To allow further analysis with respect to changing trends, the experience was broken down by the year of the primary operation. Those patients who underwent surgery before 1985 constitute the early experience; those who underwent surgery after 1986 represent the later group. The early group includes 37 patients; 18 underwent reconstruction with a nonvalved conduit, and 19 received a valved conduit. In this early group, 15 of the valved conduits were porcine, and only one homograft, an aortic, was placed. In the later group, 80 valved conduits and 23 nonvalved conduits were placed. Only one porcine valved conduit was placed in the later group, whereas 49 pulmonary and 27 aortic homografts were used.

Complications unrelated to the conduit were identified in 51

TABLE 1.
Conduits Used in Primary Operation

	TOF	PA/VSD	TGV	DORV	Truncus Arteriosus	Ross	Total
Nonvalved	1	21	7	5	7	0	41
Valved	4	23	16	8	33	15	99
Pulmonary homograft	2	9	5	3	15	15	49
Aortic homograft	2	9	3	2	13	0	28
Porcine xenograft	0	3	8	2	2	0	16
Bovine xenograft	1	2	0	1	0	0	3
Mechanical	0	0	0	0	3	0	3
Totals	5	44	23	13	40	15	140

Abbreviations: TOF, tetralogy of Fallot; *PA/VSD;* pulmonary atresia with a ventricular septal defect; *TGV,* transposition of the great double outlet right ventricle.

patients. These complications included arrhythmia in 18 patients, pulmonary hypertensive crisis in 15, bleeding requiring re-exploration in 11, and infection in 9. No patient had endocarditis during the follow-up period. The operative mortality rates are shown in Table 2. The 30-day, or in-hospital, mortality rate was 11% at the time of primary operation and was only 8% in the later group. One patient died of left ventricular failure during reoperation. Two others died later of complications not related to the conduit.

Long-term follow-up data were available for 122 patients (average follow-up, 78 months). Fifty-three reoperations have been performed; conduit failure was the reason in 41. A second reoperation (third conduit placement) was necessary in six patients, and a fourth conduit placed in two. The mean interval from initial conduit implantation to replacement was 65 months (range, 4–179 months). In the six patients who required a third conduit replacement, the mean interval was 62 months (range, 21–98 months). As seen in Table 3, those patients with complex TOF, TGV, and DORV had the greatest frequency of conduit failure, whereas those who had PA/VSD and truncus arteriosus had the least frequency. To date, no pulmonary homografts used in conjunction with the Ross procedure have required replacement in our series. In one patient in the Ross group, a 60-mm Hg gradient was observed by echocardiography 6 months after the initial procedure; the patient remains asymptomatic. Of the 41 conduit failures, stenosis was the main mode of failure in all but one. The average transconduit pressure gradient before surgery was 66 mm Hg; the gradient was as high as 106 mm Hg in one patient. After conduit replacement, the mean conduit pressure decreased by an average of 65% (range, 10% to 92%). One patient had a porcine xenograft conduit replaced because of pure regurgitation. Other reasons for replacement included

TABLE 2.
Operative Mortality Rates

	1974–1985	1986–1995	Total
Early mortality	7/37 (19%)	8/103 (8%)	15/140 (11%)
Redo mortality	0	1	1
Late mortality	0	2	2
Overall mortality	7/37 (19%)	11/103 (11%)	18/140 (13%)

TABLE 3.
Frequency of Conduit Failure

Lesion	No. of Patients (%)
Tetralogy of Fallot	3/5 (60)
Pulmonary atresia with ventricular septal defect	8/44 (18)
Transposition of great vessels	12/23 (52)
Double outlet right ventricle	7/13 (54)
Truncus arteriosus	11/40 (28)

compression of the conduit by the sternum in 1 patient, an anastomotic stenosis proximally in 1, and stenosis at the PA anastomosis or PA branch stenosis in 12. The effect of conduit type on the frequency of conduit failure is seen in Table 4. Valved conduits were significantly more likely to fail when compared with nonvalved conduits. All the porcine valve conduits in our series have been replaced. When nonvalve conduits alone were examined, Dacron conduits had a much higher failure rate than did conduits made of expanded PTFE. Among valved conduits, xenografts were more likely to fail than were homografts, and pulmonary homografts appeared to be significantly more durable than aortic homografts.

TABLE 4.
Conduit Failure

Type	No. of Procedures (%)
Nonvalved conduits	6/41 (15)
Dacron	5/20 (25)
Gortex	1/8 (13)
Impra	0/13 (0)
Valved conduits	35/99 (35)
Pulmonary homograft	5/49 (10)
Aortic homograft	10/28 (36)
Porcine	16/16 (100)
Bovine	2/3 (67)
Mechanical	2/3 (67)

RESULTS OF RIGHT VENTRICLE TO PULMONARY ARTERY CONDUIT PLACEMENT

MORTALITY RATES

Many reviews of the early, mid-, and long-term results of RV to PA conduits are available. In most larger series, more than one type of reconstruction is evaluated. This heterogeneity underscores the frustration that remains in the attempt to find the ideal conduit for a RVOT reconstruction.

The early mortality rate associated with primary conduit placement has improved over the years. In 1985, Jonas et al.[6] reported a 22% operative mortality rate among 201 patients who underwent conduit placement. Almost one half of these patients were undergoing repair of truncus arteriosus, and another 25% were undergoing the Fontan procedure. Similar results were reported 2 years later by Bull et al.[7] In that series of both homograft and heterograft conduits, the early mortality rate was approximately 30%. In 1995, Bando et al.[8] reviewed the Mayo Clinic experience of 326 patients who received cryopreserved homograft conduits. The 6% operative mortality rate in that group may have been as much related to advances in perioperative management as to the differences in the choice of conduit.

Some authors have suggested that the age at which the initial conduit placement is undertaken is a risk factor for early death. Hawkins et al.[9] reviewed the records of 89 patients who underwent placement of a cryopreserved homograft conduit from 1985 until 1990. The average age in their series was 4.3 years, and 23% of their patients were younger than 1 year of age at the time of initial conduit placement. The early mortality rates were 25% in the 20 patients younger than 1 year of age, and 2.7% in those older than 1 year.

Long-term survival also seems to be affected by early age. Bando et al.[8] reported that among patients who had an aortic homograft placed, the survival rate was significantly lower in patients younger than 4 years of age. In that study, however, young age did not affect the survival of patients who had a pulmonary homograft placed in the RVOT. A smaller conduit size index was also associated with a decreased overall survival rate. The authors show that the 5-year survival rate of patients who had undergone a previous palliative procedure was significantly improved compared with that of patients who received a homograft at the time of their initial cardiac repair. This difference appeared to be almost entirely the result of an increase in the early mortality rate in the group that underwent early definitive repair. Further multivariate analysis indicated that the presence of preoperative pulmonary hypertension was not a significant risk factor for either early or late mortality.

FACTORS INFLUENCING REOPERATION

Many investigators have also evaluated reoperation for conduit failure, or other causes. Potential sites and causes of early conduit failure include a conduit that is too small for the patient, extrinsic compression of the conduit by the sternum, and anastomotic constriction of the proximal or distal suture line. Late mechanisms include stenosis of the valve, incompetence of the valve, the development of the fibrous peel, the associated hemorrhage or thrombus formation, and the patient's outgrowing of the conduit. The effects of specific conduit types are discussed later for each type of conduit. Patient age has been identified by many as a strong predictor of reoperation. Boyce et al.[10] evaluated the long-term results of 42 patients who had a 12-mm porcine valved Dacron conduit. This conduit, which is the smallest commercially available xenograft conduit, was used to effect a complete repair during the first months of life in patients who might otherwise have undergone a palliative procedure. Twenty-eight patients underwent replacement at a mean interval of 44 months from the initial operation. Symptoms of conduit failure were present in 71% of patients. The average transconduit gradient was 83 mm Hg and was not different between symptomatic and asymptomatic patients. Boyce et al.[10] were interested in the weight gain in this group of young patients and how it affected the operation for conduit replacement. They reported a mean weight gain of 10.4 kg during the time between the initial conduit placement and reoperation. The mortality rate at reoperation was 18%. However, in the four patients whose PAs had not increased to a size that would allow placement of a conduit greater than 14 mm in diameter, the mortality rate was 75%.

Conduit replacement should be performed when symptoms appear or when RV pressures approach systemic pressure. Clinical signs of RV dysfunction, including peripheral edema, hepatic congestion, or severe atrioventricular valve regurgitation, are indications for reoperation. Unfortunately, RV dilatation and loss of systolic function can occur rapidly. Long-standing pressure overload may lead to ventricular dysfunction that is not completely reversible.[11] Several groups have noted moderate conduit obstruction without the presence of clinical symptoms.[6,12,13] Heck et al.[13] placed a catheter in 13 patients 1 year after the Rastelli procedure and found a 57% incidence of severe conduit obstruction, although symptoms were present in only 22% of the group. Stewart et al.[12] placed catheters in asymptomatic patients and observed gradients of greater than 50 mm Hg in 2 of 16 patients 1 year after surgery and in 7 of 15 patients 6 years after surgery. Diligent surveillance is obviously indicated and should be facilitated by improved echocardiographic techniques.

In 1984, Schaff et al.[14] reviewed the results of 100 consecutive operations for replacement of RV to PA conduits. Among the patients in this series, the mean age at reoperation was 13 years. The operative mortality rate was 7%, but no operative deaths occurred among the 47 patients who required only conduit replacement without repair of another defect.

Bando et al.[8] reported that calcification and obstruction of aortic homografts were significantly greater in patients younger than 4 years of age when compared with older patients. In the same study, only 4% of pulmonary homografts became stenotic, but almost all had been implanted in patients older than 4 years of age. The predisposition to calcification of aortic homografts is discussed below. Bando et al.[8] showed that, in the younger age group, the diagnoses of truncus arteriosus, TGV, and DORV were associated with a higher rate of homograft failure.

SPECIFIC CONDUIT TYPES

Valved vs. Nonvalved Conduits

Concerns regarding the long-term durability of xenograft valves, and the desire to avoid anticoagulation, have led to an interest in the use of nonvalved extracardiac conduits for RVOT reconstruction. Worries regarding RV failure in patients who have a nonvalved conduit in the long-term, however, have limited their use. This type of repair, which is applicable only to patients who do not have pulmonary hypertension, has been commonly used in the repair of TOF for many years. Dacron, expanded PTFE, and autologous and bovine pericardium have all been used in this type of repair. In our series of 140 conduit placements, only 41 nonvalve conduits have been placed as an initial procedure, and most were placed before 1985. Our group has developed an animal model to evaluate right heart conduit performance and durability.[15, 16] Neointimal hyperplasia develops quicker in Dacron conduits tested in this model (3–6 months) than in human beings, but remains similar in distribution and histologic appearance to what is identified clinically (Fig 3). Using this model, we evaluated porcine valved and nonvalved Dacron conduits in dogs and found a threefold increase in the thickness of the neointimal lining of the valved conduits.[15] In the valved conduits, the peel was fenestrated and poorly adherent to the Dacron conduit, as has been observed clinically.[18] We postulate that this thick neointima accumulates as a result of the low pressure phasic flow through the right heart and that the omission of the valve allows a to-and-fro washing motion in the nonvalved conduits. For the past 10 years, only non-Dacron, nonvalved conduits have been used. We have preferred a stented expanded PTFE conduit to minimize both neointimal formation and compression of the conduit by surrounding structures (Fig 4).

Xenograft Valve Conduits

The use of bovine pericardial conduits for RVOT reconstruction has been sporadic, and much less is known about the behavior of these conduits than about the more common porcine valved conduits. Agarwal et al.[17, 18] have extensively evaluated the pathogenesis and mechanism of failure of porcine valved Dacron conduits. Failure can be further subdivided into either valvar- or conduit-related mechanisms. Placement of too small of a valve will result

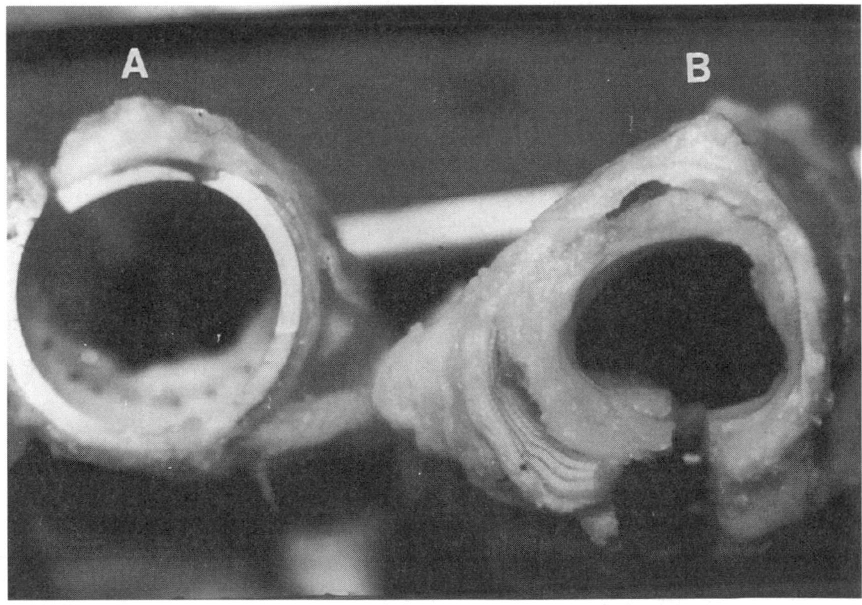

FIGURE 3.

Experimental right ventricle to pulmonary artery conduits. **A,** expanded polytetrafluoroethylene conduit with minimal neointimal peel. **B,** Dacron valved conduit with thick, loosely attached neointimal peel.

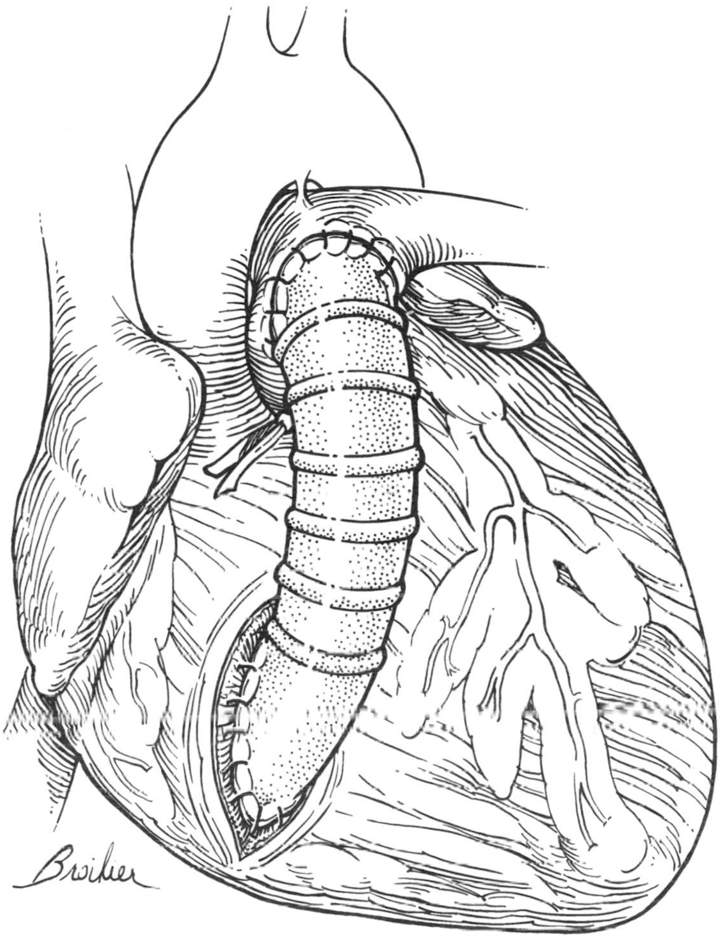

FIGURE 4.
A nonvalved right ventricle to pulmonary artery conduit constructed with the use of a ringed expanded polytetrafluoroethylene graft. (Courtesy of Brown JW: *J Thorac Cardiovasc Surg* 90:835, 1985.)

in early inherent stenosis. Smaller porcine valves may have an initial gradient as high as 25 mm Hg,[17] for which the inherent muscular ridge present in the porcine aortic valve used in commercially available Dacron valved conduits is largely responsible. Acquired valve failure can occur through calcification, thrombosis, or incompetence. Calcification is a common mode of failure in porcine xenografts used not only as extracardiac conduits but also in the orthotopic position; this failure is more frequent in children.[31] It usually begins as mineralization of the retained aortic remnant close to the commissures and progresses to involve the commissures until they become fixed.[17] Severely stenotic valves will also often possess nodular calcific excrescences throughout the cusp tissue. Thrombus formation is always associated with the calcification and disruption of the cusp tissue, although it remains unclear whether this thrombosis antecedes or precedes calcification.[17] As the cusps become fixed, incompetence results from the lack of coaptation. Tears also occur in the cusps because of calcification. In addition, infection secondary to endocarditis leads to destruction and incompetence of the valve cusp.

A thick neointimal fibrous peel is present in most explanted Dacron conduits. Unlike conduits placed in the systemic circulation, this peel is poorly adherent to the graft material and is characterized by fenestrations that allow a layer of thrombus to form between the conduit and the peel.[17] Development and progression of this thrombus causes luminal obstruction. Catastrophic acute conduit obstruction has occasionally been reported as a result of this phenomenon.[17] Dacron grafts have performed poorly as venous substitutes.[19, 20] To alleviate these problems, our group has investigated the use of an externally stented PTFE valved conduit.[21] As an RV to PA conduit material, externally stented PTFE conduits had only one fourth the neointimal peel seen on woven or knitted Dacron conduits. Similarly, there was less degradation of the porcine heterograft valves in the stented PTFE conduits (Fig 5). In the animal model, the neointimal peel seemed to migrate into the sinuses of the porcine valves, thereby restricting their mobility.[21]

Homografts

Ross and Somerville[3] first proposed the use of aortic homografts to reconstruct the RVOT in 1966. Since then, the use of these grafts has been met with varying enthusiasm. Homografts sterilized with irradiation failed early and were largely abandoned. Even though there was some information as early 1976 that cryopreservation or cold storage of these grafts would improve their long-term function,[22] the more readily available porcine valved xenograft conduits were used with greater frequency in this country. Continued improvements in the cryopreservation techniques and in the proliferation of organ procurement programs and tissue banks provided a renewed interest in homografts for use in reconstruction of many complex congenital lesions, including RVOT reconstruction. Homografts offer many theoretical and practical benefits over xenografts: Anticoagulation is not needed; excellent hemodynamic performance can be achieved, especially in smaller sizes; and some of the technical aspects of the procedure are easier to effect, particularly in infants and small children.

Initially, aortic homografts were favored because the aortic tissue is thicker and less friable than the thinner PA tissue. It was also believed that aortic valves and aortic tissue might withstand high right-sided pressures better in patients with pulmonary hypertension. The available aortic length is also greater than the available PA length for any given valve size, thereby eliminating the need for extension of the distal conduit. Kirklin et al.[23] reviewed the fate of 147 aortic valve homografts implanted for RVOT reconstruction between 1981 and 1986. These results were compared with those of two earlier groups of patients in whom irradiated or glutaraldehyde-preserved allografts or porcine xenograft conduit reconstructions had been used for the same purpose. In the study group, the mean interval between operation and follow-up was 27 months. In the comparison groups, the mean follow-up was 9 years. Two of the cryopreserved valves were replaced because of obstruction 28 and 42 months after the initial implantation. An additional 24 patients underwent postoperative cardiac catheterization; all

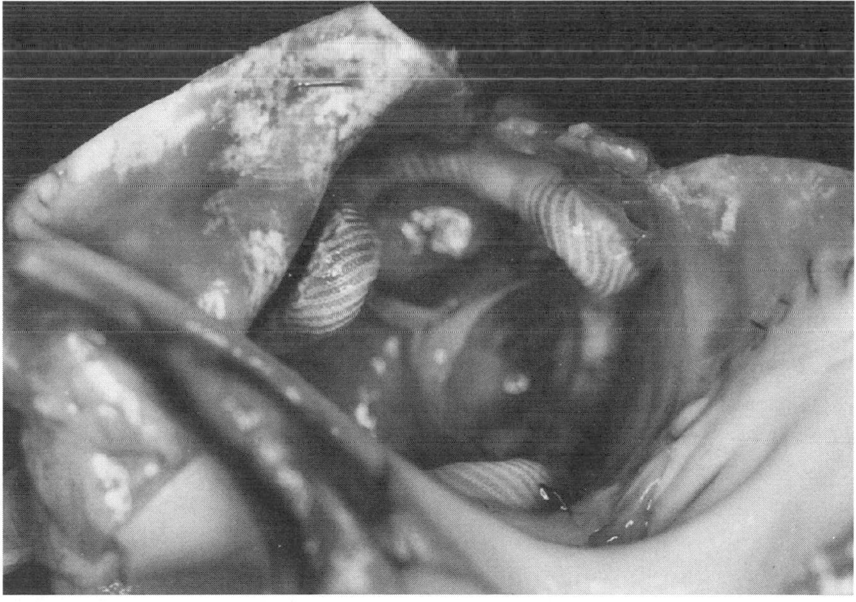

FIGURE 5.

An explanted (6 months) expanded polytetrafluoroethylene conduit that contains a porcine xenograft. Note the lack of neointimal peel.

these patients had a gradient of more than 40 mm Hg across the conduit. In three patients, the obstruction appeared to be within the homograft, whereas in two it was determined to be at the distal anastomosis. On the basis of these early results, Kirklin et al.[23] speculated that if a large enough homograft were used, a complete and permanent repair might be possible in children aged 3–5 years. Other investigators have also noted that larger sized homografts appeared to perform better. Tan et al.[24] reported the results of 45 patients whose status was followed a mean of 8.6 years after RVOT reconstruction with an antibiotic preserved aortic homograft. Only four patients required reoperation for conduit stenosis. The age (mean, 35 days) and weight (median, 4 kg) of these patients were similar to those of patients reported by Heineman et al,[25] (mean age, 34 days; mean weight, 3.4 kg). However, the median size of the homograft used by Tan et al. was 15.6 mm, compared with the homografts of 7–13 mm used by Heinemann et al. Several other patients in this series had calcification in the wall of the aortic homograft but did not have evidence of obstruction. This finding was again attributed to the use of a larger sized homograft. Many authors have also suggested that the age at the time of implantation affects the long-term function of aortic homograft and the RVOT. In the report from the Mayo Clinic, 26% of aortic homografts in patients younger than 4 years of age became stenotic, compared with only 11% in the group older than 4 years of age.[8] This group also noted that the type of homograft was the strongest predictor of homograft failure and believed that pulmonary homografts represented the best conduit available at this time for RVOT reconstruction. There are several theoretical advantages to the pulmonary homograft. The PA tissue is a better match for the native PA than is the thicker aortic tissue. The bifurcated pulmonary homograft can also be used to augment or even replace stenotic or atretic branch PAs. Albert et al.[26] showed similar survival statistics but better hemodynamic performance for cryopreserved pulmonary homografts compared with aortic homografts or porcine valved conduits. Unfortunately, a later report from the same institution showed that, in children younger than 1 year of age at the time of implantation, fibrocalcific degradation was being identified with increasing frequency.[27] Several mechanisms have been proposed, including increased elastin and calcium content in aortic homografts compared with pulmonary homografts.

The effect of immunologic mechanisms on homograft survival continues to be investigated. Balch and Karp[28] showed no effect of ABO type on homograft aortic valves placed in a freehand method of aortic valve replacement. Bando et al.[8] also showed no effect of ABO matching on homograft survival. However, many groups, including ours, still prefer to match donor and recipient ABO group whenever possible. The differences in conduit survival between older and younger patient groups has also been attributed to immunologic mechanisms. Because the percentage of circulating CD5+B (B1) cells to CD5−B cells and T cells is high at birth and decreases with age, and because human B1 cells produce a generalized immune response whereas CD5−B and T cells produce a more specific antigenic response, Clarke and Bishop[27] have speculated that the more immunologically immature infant may mount a more generalized attack against viable allograft tissue. Lupinetti et al.[29] have shown the association between the immune system and calcification of allografts in an animal model.

"Poor" preservation, or handling techniques, may also have a beneficial effect on homograft survival, by decreasing the number of viable endothelial cells. Clarke and Bishop[27] speculated that improved survival in homografts greater than 20 mm in diameter might have been secondary to the placement of the surgeon's finger within the graft while trimming it before insertion. Similarly Basket et al.[30] have recently suggested that an interval of longer than 24 hours from the time of homograft retrieval until cryopreservation was associated with improved echocardiographic performance. Shorter intervals have been correlated with improved endothelial viability, which again may suggest an immunologic basis for homograft dysfunction. Others have speculated that administration of nonsteroidal anti-inflammatory agents, or even low-dose cyclosporine, decreases the immunologic response. Our current practice is to treat all homograft recipients with therapeutic doses of ibuprofen (5 mg/kg 4 times per day).

When a pulmonary homograft has been used to reconstruct the RVOT as part of the Ross procedure, similar conduit deterioration has not been identified.[32] Several reasons for this improved function have been proposed, but the most important reason may have to do with the placement of the valve in the orthotopic position. We speculate that this approach improves the flow characteristics across the valve, thereby leading to fewer areas of stasis and fewer areas of turbulence.

REFERENCES

1. Kinner W, Zenker R: Experience with correction of Fallot's tetralogy in 178 cases. *Surgery* 57:353–357, 1965.
2. Rastelli GC, Ongley PA, David GD, et al: Surgical repair for pulmo-

nary valve atresia with coronary-pulmonary artery failure: Report of a case. *Mayo Clin Proc* 40:521–527, 1965.

3. Ross DN, Sommerville J: Correction of pulmonary atresia with a homograft aortic valve. *Lancet* 2:1446–1447, 1966.
4. Bowman FO Jr, Hancock WD, Malm JR: A valve containing Dacron prosthesis: Its use for restoring pulmonary artery–right ventricular continuity. *Arch Surg* 107:724–728, 1973.
5. Kirklin JW, Barrett-Boyes BG: *Cardiac Surgery,* ed 2. New York, Wiley, 1993, p 560, Appendix 12-A.
6. Jonas RA, Freed MD, Mayer JE, et al: Long term follow-up of patients with synthetic right heart conduits. *Circulation* 72:77S–83S, 1985.
7. Bull C, MacCartney FJ, Horvath P, et al: Evaluation of long term results of homograft and heterograft valves in extra cardiac conduits. *J Thorac Cardiovasc Surg* 94:12–19, 1987.
8. Bando K, Danielson GK, Schaff HV, et al: Outcome of pulmonary and aortic homografts for right ventricular outflow tract reconstruction. *J Thorac Cardiovasc Surg* 109:509–518, 1995.
9. Hawkins JA, Bailey WW, Dillon T, et al: Midterm results with cryopreserved allograft conduits from the right ventricle to the pulmonary arteries. *J Thorac Cardiovasc Surg* 104:910–915, 1992.
10. Boyce SW, Turly K, Yee ES, et al: The fate of the 12 mm porcine valved conduit from the right ventricle to the pulmonary artery. *J Thorac Cardiovasc Surg* 95:201–207, 1988.
11. Sano S, Karl TR, Mee RB: Extracardiac valved conduits in the pulmonary circuit. *Ann Thorac Surg* 52:285–290, 1991.
12. Stewart S, Maning J, Alexson C, et al: The Hancock external valved conduit. A dichotomy between late clinical results and late cardiac catheterization findings. *J Thorac Cardiovasc Surg* 86:562–569, 1983.
13. Heck HA Jr, Schieken RM, Lauer RM, et al: Conduit repair for complex congenital heart disease. Late follow up. *Thorac Cardiovasc Surg* 75:806–814, 1978.
14. Schaff HV, DiDonato RM, Danielson GK, et al: Reoperation for obstructed pulmonary ventricle–pulmonary artery conduits. *J Thorac Cardiovasc Surg* 88:334–343, 1984.
15. Fiore AC, Peigh PS, Robinson RJ, et al: Valved and nonvalved right ventricular–pulmonary arterial extracardiac conduits. *J Thorac Cardiovasc Surg* 86:490–497, 1983.
16. Fiore AC, Peigh PS, Sears NJ, et al: The prevention of extracardiac conduit obstruction: An experimental study. *J Surg Res* 34:463–472, 1983.
17. Agarwal KC, Edwards WD, Feldt RH, et al: Clinicopathological correlates of obstructed right sided porcine valved extracardiac conduits. *J Thorac Cardiovasc Surg* 81:591–601, 1981.
18. Agarwal KC, Edwards WD, Feldt RH, et al: Pathogenesis of nonobstructive fibrous peels in porcine valved extracardiac conduits. *J Thorac Cardiovasc Surg* 83:584–589, 1982.
19. Robison RJ, Peigh PS, Fiore AC, et al: Venous prostheses: Improved patency with external stents. *J Surg Res* 36:306–311, 1984.

20. Fiore AC, Brown JW, Concirtie RS, et al: Prosthetic replacement of the thoracic vena cava. *J Thorac Cardiovasc Surg* 84:560–568, 1982.
21. Brown JW, Halpin MP, Rescorla FJ, et al: Externally stented polytetrafluoroethylene valved conduits for right heart reconstruction. *J Thorac Cardiovasc Surg* 90:833–841, 1983.
22. Angell JD, Christopher BS, Hawtrey O, et al: A fresh viable human heart valve bank: Sterilization, sterility testing, and cryogenic preservation. *Transplant Proc* 8:139S–147S, 1967.
23. Kirklin JW, Blackstone EH, Maehara T, et al: Intermediate-term fate of cryopreserved allograft and xenograft valved conduits. *Ann Thorac Surg* 44:598–606, 1987.
24. Tan RK, Tolan MJ, Zamvar VY, et al: Use of larger sized aortic homograft conduits in right ventricular outflow tract reconstruction. *J Heart Valve Dis* 4:660–664, 1995.
25. Heinemann MK, Hanley FL, Fenton KN, et al: Fate of small homograft conduits after early repair of truncus arteriosus. *Ann Thorac Surg* 55:1409–1412, 1993.
26. Albert JD, Bishop DA, Fulerton DA, et al: Conduit reconstruction of the right ventricular outflow tract. *J Thorac Cardiovasc Surg* 106:228–236, 1993.
27. Clarke DR, Bishop DA: Ten year experience with pulmonary allografts in children. *J Heart Valve Dis* 4:384–391, 1995.
28. Balch CM, Karp RB: Blood group compatibility and aortic valve allotransplantation in man. *J Thorac Cardiovasc Surg* 70:256–259, 1975.
29. Lupinetti FM, Cobb KC, Kioshcos HC, et al: Effect of immunological differences on rat aortic valve allograft calcification. *J Cardiac Surg* 7:65-70, 1992.
30. Basket RJ, Ross DB, Nanton MA, et al: Factors in the early failure of cryopreserved homograft pulmonary valves in children: Preserved immunogenicity? Presented at the American Association For Thoracic Surgery, San Diego, Calif, May 1996.
31. Dunn JM: Porcine valve durability in children. *Ann Thorac Surg* 32:357–368, 1981.
32. The Ross Procedure. *International Registry Annual Summary Report,* April 1996.

Lung Transplantation in Children

Nancy D. Bridges, M.D.
Assistant Professor of Pediatrics (Cardiology), University of Pennsylvania School of Medicine; Medical Director, Lung and Heart/Lung Transplantation and Pulmonary Hypertension Services, Children's Hospital of Philadelphia

Thomas L. Spray, M.D.
Professor of Surgery, University of Pennsylvania School of Medicine; Chief, Cardiothoracic Surgery and Director, Thoracic Organ Transplantation, Children's Hospital of Philadelphia

---

Experience with single or bilateral lung transplantation in children, especially preadolescent children, remains limited. The 1995 St. Louis International Lung Transplant Registry records a total of 374 lung transplant procedures in children younger than 16 years of age; of these, 38 were performed in patients who had cardiovascular disease, and the remainder in patients who had parenchymal pulmonary disease.[1] The pediatric lung transplant program at Children's Hospital of Philadelphia deals with a unique population composed primarily, although not exclusively, of children who have cardiovascular disease and whose who have been rejected by other programs because of "high-risk" characteristics. In this chapter, we discuss our approach to pediatric lung transplantation.

Lung transplantation in children must be considered a palliative procedure, the long-term outcome of which remains quite uncertain for the individual patient. The social, emotional, and financial implications of lung transplantation for the patient and family are enormous. We find the following strategies useful in reducing the stress for families: education about the realities of lung transplantation before their commitment to the procedure; minimization of barriers to lung transplantation, such as arbitrary "absolute contraindications"; acceptance of outside studies whenever possible in the evaluation of transplant candidates; limitation of pretransplant testing to those studies that will truly have an impact on decision-making and assessment of risk; minimization of arbitrary protocols relating to pre- or post-transplant testing and manage-

© 1996, Mosby–Year Book, Inc.

ment; and cooperation and communication with local physicians to allow patients to spend as much time as possible at home.

PATIENT SELECTION AND TIMING OF LISTING

All children who are being considered for lung transplantation must have end-stage pulmonary or cardiovascular disease with a predicted 2-year survival probability of 50% or less. This criterion is based on the current predicted 2-year survival of 60% among children undergoing lung transplantation.[2] In addition, alternative therapies for their condition must be proved ineffective or nonexistent. The time of listing is, in theory, determined by the predicted duration of survival without transplantation and predicted waiting times for lungs, neither of which is known with certainty.

PATIENT SELECTION AND TIMING OF LISTING FOR PATIENTS WHO HAVE PULMONARY DISEASE

The single most common diagnosis among children undergoing lung transplantation is cystic fibrosis.[1] Aggressive management of this disease, however, has resulted in preservation of adequate lung function into late adolescence and adulthood, so that cystic fibrosis is an uncommon indication for lung transplantation in preadolescent children. Medical evaluation and criteria for listing of adolescents with cystic fibrosis are essentially the same as in adults. Pulmonary function testing and clinical course are the most important prognostic factors in these patients; listing for transplantation generally can be considered when the forced expiratory volume in 1 second decreases to less than 30% of predicted.[3] Frequent recurrent pulmonary infection and increasing frequency of hospitalization may also be considered indicators of deterioration. These factors must be considered in the timing of listing, especially if the waiting time is expected to be long. Colonization of the airways or sinuses with *Pseudomonas* species, which are pan-resistant to single or synergistic antibiotics, is not an absolute contraindication to lung transplantation in our program.

Other pulmonary diagnoses that lead to lung transplantation in children include idiopathic pulmonary fibrosis, surfactant protein B deficiency, bronchopulmonary dysplasia, bronchiolitis obliterans, and a variety of other conditions; the overall mix is considerably more heterogeneous than in the adult population.[4] Pulmonary diagnoses for which lung transplantation has been performed at our center are shown in Table 1. For some conditions, such as surfactant protein B deficiency, the absence of effective medical therapy and severely limited life span justify listing for transplantation at the time of diagnosis. For others, such as bron-

TABLE 1.
Diagnoses for Which Lung Transplantation Has Been Performed at Children's Hospital of Philadelphia

All patients underwent bilateral sequential lung transplantation performed with cardiopulmonary bypass

Pulmonary diagnoses: Primary lung transplants
- OB 2° to graft-vs.-host disease, after bone marrow transplantation for Wiskott-Aldrich syndrome
- Severe cystic bronchopulmonary dysplasia, after partial right pneumonectomy
- Cystic fibrosis

Pulmonary diagnoses: Repeat lung transplants
- Graft failure 2° to adenovirus pneumonia
- OB after heart and lung transplantation for PHT in association with transposition of the great arteries, after arterial switch procedure
- Graft failure 2° to presumed viral pneumonitis and aspiration pneumonia
- Graft failure 2° to graft vasculopathy

Cardiovascular diagnoses:
- PHT in association with transposition of the great arteries, after Mustards' operation; concurrent repair of atrial baffle leaks
- PHT in association with critical coarctation of the aorta, after repair of coarctation of the aorta
- Pulmonary veno-occlusive disease
- Primary PHT; concurrent repair of atrial septal defect
- Congenital pulmonary vein stenosis; concurrent repair of atrial septal defect
- PHT in association with partial anomalous pulmonary venous return, portal hypertension, and hypersplenism; concurrent repair of partial anomalous pulmonary venous return and atrial septal defect, concurrent splenectomy

Abbreviations: OB, obliterative bronchiolitis; *PHT,* pulmonary hypertension.

chopulmonary dysplasia, the wide variability in the course of the disease and potential for recovery of the native lung mandate an individualized approach to potential candidates.

PATIENT SELECTION AND TIMING OF LISTING FOR PATIENTS WHO HAVE CARDIOVASCULAR DISEASE

Cardiovascular diagnoses leading to lung transplantation in children may be divided into three broad categories: pulmonary hypertension without congenital heart disease (most often, primary pulmonary hypertension), pulmonary hypertension in association with congenital heart disease, and inadequate pulmonary vascular bed.[5] Cardiovascular diagnoses for which lung transplantation, with or without cardiac repair, has been performed at our center are shown in Table 1. All children with a cardiovascular diagnoses who are evaluated for lung transplantation undergo cardiac catheterization for drug testing and disease staging. A subset of patients who have primary pulmonary hypertension will respond to and live longer as a result of treatment with pulmonary vasodilators, such as calcium channel blocking agents and prostacyclin[6, 7]; anticoagulation also appears to prolong survival.[6] We administer vasodilators chronically whenever there is a positive or neutral response to the acute administration of these agents in the cardiac catheterization laboratory.

Given the current prognosis for children undergoing lung transplantation (approximately 60% survival at 2 years), timing of transplantation is a crucial and troublesome issue in those who have pulmonary hypertension of any form. There are few available data regarding survival of children who have primary or secondary pulmonary hypertension. The National Institutes of Health study of survival in adults who have primary pulmonary hypertension is frequently cited in this regard.[8] Two recent studies in children, one limited to those with primary pulmonary hypertension[9] and one including those with either the primary or secondary form of pulmonary hypertension,[10] indicate that hemodynamic parameters are important predictors of survival, thereby justifying invasive study of patients being evaluated for transplantation. We use the product of the right atrial pressure and the indexed pulmonary vascular resistance as a guide for listing patients who have pulmonary hypertension. For example, in a child whose pulmonary vascular resistance is 18 Wood's units indexed and whose right atrial pressure is 14 mm Hg, the product of these two numbers is 252 mm $Hg^2/min/m^2/L^{-1}$. As is shown in Figure 1, a child in whom the product of right atrial pressure and pulmonary vascular resistance (measured in indexed Wood's units) is greater than 160 has a significantly better 2-year survival with lung transplantation than without. In the case of congenital pulmonary vein stenosis or pulmonary veno-occlusive disease, lung transplantation is the only treatment associated with even medium-term survival[11] (Fig 2); we believe that these children should be listed for lung transplantation at the time of diagnosis. Medical management with vasodilators, along with palliative dilation or stenting of the pulmonary veins, may help a child who has pulmonary vein stenosis survive until organs become available.

Patients who have end-stage pulmonary hypertension are hemodynamically quite fragile; medical treatment of such children presents a considerable challenge. In our experience, the diagnosis of pulmonary hypertension, without an anatomical communication to permit right to left shunting, is associated with a mortality rate of up to 46% while waiting for organs.[12] Death results from progressive right heart failure, which culminates in an acute bradycardic event. We have occasionally been successful in resuscitating such patients by avoiding the administration of epinephrine and using large doses of isoproterenol, followed by stabilization with extracorporeal membrane oxygenation (ECMO); in our experience, however, the use of ECMO after cardiac arrest in these patients has not resulted in successful lung transplantation. Rather, ECMO as a bridge to transplantation is most likely to be successful when used electively, before cardiac arrest. Elective transcatheter creation of an atrial septal defect has been shown to prolong sur-

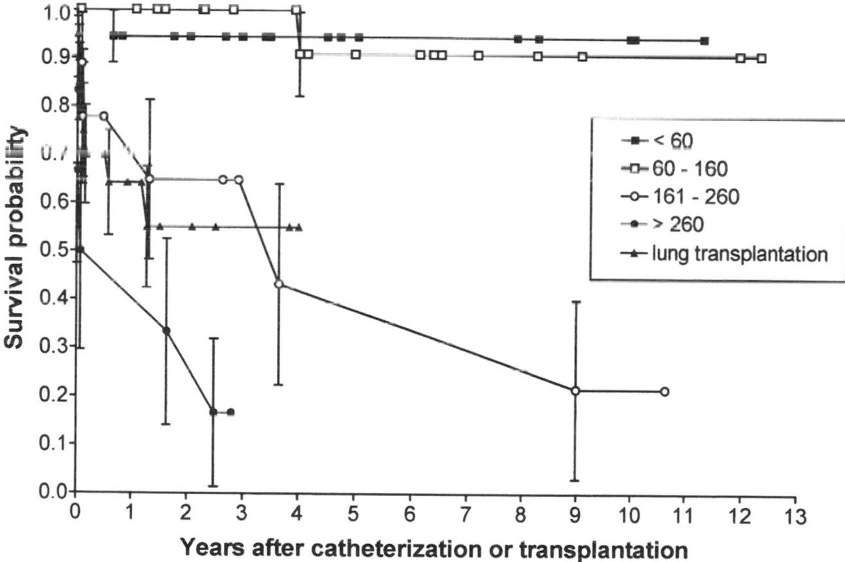

FIGURE 1.

Survival probability for patients with primary or secondary pulmonary hypertension, with and without lung transplant. Patients who did not undergo transplantation are stratified by the product of their mean right atrial pressure (in mm Hg) and their pulmonary vascular resistance (in Wood's units). For example, for a patient with a right atrial pressure of 8 mm Hg and a pulmonary vascular resistance of 6 Wood's units, this product equals 48.

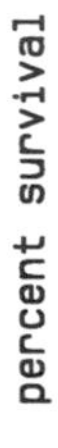

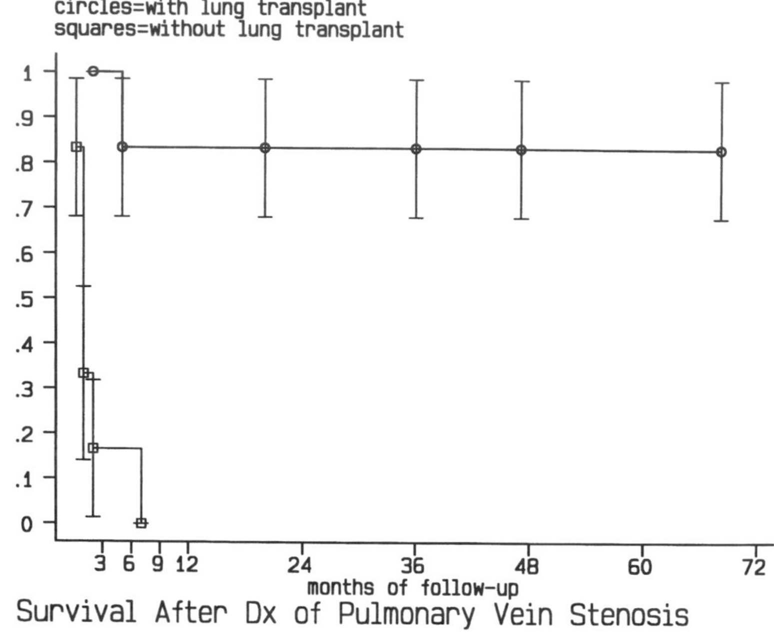

FIGURE 2.
Actuarial survival after diagnosis of pulmonary vein stenosis. Note that lung transplantation is the only treatment associated with even medium-term survival.

vival in patients who have end-stage pulmonary hypertension and elevated right atrial pressure.[13]

CHOICE OF TRANSPLANT PROCEDURE

LUNG VS. HEART-LUNG TRANSPLANT

Whenever there is adequate left ventricular performance and cardiac valve competence, we generally prefer lung transplantation with concurrent cardiac repair to heart and lung transplantation. This procedure allows for better use of donor organs, because hearts are then available for those patients who have no reconstructive alternative. In addition, the lung recipient is spared the threat of post-transplant coronary artery disease or cardiac rejection. Even when repair of a cardiac lesion requires use of a prosthetic conduit, as in tetralogy of Fallot with pulmonary atresia, the durability of the cardiac repair will probably exceed that of the transplanted lungs. Given the scarcity of heart-lung blocks, we predict that more complex cardiac lesions will be repaired in association with lung transplantation in the future. Cardiac repairs performed concurrently with lung transplantation in our program in St. Louis and subsequently in Philadelphia are shown in Table 2.

SINGLE VS. BILATERAL LUNG TRANSPLANT; LIVING-RELATED LUNG TRANSPLANT

In most cases, we prefer to perform bilateral lung transplantation, particularly in very young patients. In these patients, the total parenchymal mass of a single lung will be quite small, and its growth potential as yet is unknown. We have performed bilateral transplantation of lobes from a larger donor when size-matched organs were not available. We have also used lobes from living-related donors (a lower lobe from each of two adult donors) in critically ill children who seemed certain to die before cadaveric lungs became available. Living-related lobar donation is in general practical only for recipients 95–100 cm or more in length, because of the size of an adult lobe. We consider living-related lung transplantation a good alternative for selected patients, i.e., those who have been listed for lung transplantation and whose condition has deteriorated to the point that they are unlikely to survive until organs become available by the current methods of allocation. Examples of appropriate candidates for living-related lung transplantation

TABLE 2.
Cardiac Repairs Performed Concurrently With Single or Bilateral Lung Transplantation

Suture closure of patent ductus arteriosus
Division of vascular ring
Suture closure of atrial septal defect
Patch closure of ventricular septal defect
Reconstruction of previously ligated pulmonary artery
Repair of partial anomalous pulmonary venous return
Reconstruction of pulmonary venous confluence in congenital pulmonary vein stenosis or pulmonary veno-occlusive disease
Repair of baffle leaks in a patient with D-transposition of the great arteries, after Mustards' operation
Repair of double chambered right ventricle/ventricular septal defect: Patch closure of ventricular septal defect, excision of right ventricular muscle bundles, pericardial patch enlargement of the right ventricular outflow tract
Repair of tetralogy of Fallot with pulmonary atresia: Patch closure of ventricular septal defect, right ventricular outflow tract construction with homograft to reconstructed pulmonary confluence

would include children with cystic fibrosis who require intubation and mechanical ventilation and children with pulmonary vascular disease who require support with ECMO. Bilateral lung transplantation is usually considered necessary in patients who have septic lung disease (i.e., cystic fibrosis) to prevent contamination of the transplanted lung with organisms harbored in the contralateral lung; however, successful single lung transplantation with contralateral pneumonectomy has been reported in this setting.[14] Single lung transplantation is associated with a greater degree of postoperative hemodynamic instability, particularly in patients with pulmonary hypertension, in whom the entire cardiac output will go to the transplanted lung after surgery. In addition, single lung transplantation necessarily leaves the patient with less pulmonary reserve than would bilateral lung transplantation. Nevertheless, single lung transplantation has been associated with excellent long-term outcomes; in some settings, it may be the preferred lung transplant procedure. In children who have had previous thoracic operations, avoidance of the previously entered thorax may be desirable. In those patients who may have some potential for lung recovery, single lung transplantation can be considered an alternative to long-term ECMO as a "bridge" to recovery of the contralateral lung.

HIGH-RISK CHARACTERISTICS IN PEDIATRIC LUNG TRANSPLANT CANDIDATES: DO WE KNOW WHAT THEY ARE?

As experience with lung transplantation has increased, so has acceptance of high-risk candidates for the procedure. Among 14 patients who have undergone lung or heart-lung transplantation at our institution, high-risk characteristics have been the rule rather than the exception, as shown in Table 3. Nevertheless, we have had only one early death, which occurred in a child who had a second lung transplant after losing her first graft at 6 months to graft vasculopathy; she died of invasive aspergillosis 2 weeks after the second transplant. All 13 of our survivors are at home and enjoying a functional status that is significantly better than their pretransplant state. We therefore believe that consideration of individual patient characteristics can permit lung transplantation in most children, and arbitrary contraindications should not be considered absolute.

ISSUES AFTER SUCCESSFUL LUNG TRANSPLANTATION

OBLITERATIVE BRONCHIOLITIS

Obliterative bronchiolitis (OB) remains the most important barrier to long-term survival after lung transplantation. Among children

TABLE 3.
High-risk Characteristics Among Children Undergoing Lung Transplantation at Children's Hospital of Philadelphia, December 1994 to January 1996

Characteristics	No. of Patients (%)
Previous thoracotomy and/or sternotomy	11/14 (79)
Previous lung transplant	4/14 (29)
Concurrent cardiac repair	6/14 (43)
Mechanical ventilation lasting > 7 days just before transplant	7/14 (50)
Tracheostomy	5/14 (36)
Extracorporeal membrane oxygenation	1/14 (7)
Debilitation or inability to ambulate	8/14 (57)
Serious disease of other organ systems*	3/14 (21)

*Portal hypertension with hypersplenism requiring splenectomy at the time of lung transplantation, one patient; Wiskott-Aldrich syndrome treated with bone marrow transplantation with graft-vs.-host disease, one patient; and tracheo-esophageal fistula, repaired, with severe gastrointestinal dysmotility and recurrent pancreatitis, one patient.

who have undergone lung transplantation in St. Louis and Philadelphia, OB has been diagnosed in 26% and has contributed to two thirds of late deaths. Interestingly, in our experience OB has (so far) been absent among children who underwent transplant before the age of 3 years, which suggests that the patient's immunologic history may play a role in the development of OB. Although the etiology and pathophysiology of this process remain elusive, the condition most consistently associated with OB is cytomegalovirus infection. At Children's Hospital of Philadelphia, we administer gancyclovir for 6 weeks as prophylaxis in all lung transplant recipients after transplantation, regardless of the serologic status of either the donor or the recipient, to reduce the risk of early cytomegalovirus infection at a time when infection is most serious.

INFECTION WITH UBIQUITOUS VIRUSES

Patients who undergo lung transplantation at a young age are more likely to have their first encounter with common viruses (e.g., adenovirus, parainfluenza, influenza, Epstein-Barr virus, and respiratory syncytial virus) in an immunocompromised state. The results of such an encounter can be devastating. In our experience, infection with adenovirus or parainfluenza virus has been the most common cause of death or graft failure in patients younger than 2 years of age who undergo lung transplantation,[15] and primary Epstein-Barr virus infection is associated with the development of post-transplant lymphoproliferative disease.[16] On the other hand, respiratory syncytial virus appears to be well tolerated, albeit associated with prolonged antigen positivity.

REJECTION

Acute vascular rejection has been an uncommon occurrence in our experience, perhaps because of the age of our patient population. For patients who are tolerating their grafts well more than 3 months after transplantation, we are relatively aggressive in reducing the level of immunosuppression in hopes of reducing the incidence and severity of viral infections, especially in our youngest patients. We, like others, have found that tacrolimus may be used successfully in the treatment of rejection that has been unresponsive to cyclosporin. Tacrolimus has other advantages as well. In very young patients, we have found that the gingival hypertrophy associated with cyclosporin makes tooth emergence very difficult; this problem is resolved when patients are treated with tacrolimus. In addition, the cosmetic consequences of treatment with cyclosporin are quite serious in some patients. Our current immunosuppressive regimen is given in Table 4.

TABLE 4.
Immunosuppression for Lung Transplantation at Children's Hospital of Philadelphia

During the immediate postoperative period:
- Cyclosporin by continuous infusion to maintain a blood level of 300–350 μg/L
- Azathioprine, 2 mg/kg IV daily
- Methylprednisolone, 1 mg/kg IV daily

Once enteral medications can be given:
- Tacrolimus initially given twice a day to maintain a blood level of 10–15 ng/mL; the dosage is reduced as tolerated to a blood level of 5–10 ng/mL.
- Azathioprine, 2 mg/kg/day, or mycophenolate mofetil, 15 mg/kg twice a day
- Prednisolone, 1 mg/kg daily, reduced as tolerated to 0.3 mg/kg every other day

GROWTH, DEVELOPMENT, AND FUNCTIONAL STATUS

Data are scarce with regard to growth and development. Our experience, both in Philadelphia and in St. Louis, is that most children are within normal limits in terms of stature and growth velocity after lung transplantation but tend to be at the lower end of the normal range.[15]

TECHNICAL ISSUES

The technical aspects of lung transplantation in children have been addressed in previous studies.[4] Transplantation is generally performed with the use of cardiopulmonary bypass in children because it facilitates the removal of both lungs and cardiac repair. Both lungs are also removed in patients who have primary pulmonary disease with the patient supported on cardiopulmonary bypass. This procedure allows the anesthesiologist to irrigate the trachea with antibiotics in patients who have septic lung disease to prevent contamination of the transplanted lungs. It also decreases the ischemic time on the second implant, because dissection and removal of the second lung is not required before implantation. We have not noted complications from the use of cardiopulmonary bypass in our patients. In addition, the use of cardiopulmonary bypass routinely permits repair of cardiac defects before implantation of the donor lungs and prevents the need for the entire cardiac output to pass through the first transplanted lung, which may cause early congestion of the lung and hemodynamic instability.

The primary concern in children is bronchial anastomotic complications and growth of the airways. We perform primary end-to-end anastomoses of the bronchus bilaterally with the bilateral sequential technique to allow for the best vascularization of the airways. This approach has resulted in the lowest incidence of airway complication in our larger series from St. Louis. From July 1990 to April 1994, 49 patients undergoing 51 transplants with 98 bronchial anastomoses were evaluated for dehiscence or stenosis.[17] Risk factors, including age, size, pretransplant diagnosis, airway organisms and technique of bronchial anastomosis, donor ischemic time, and presence of rejection, were evaluated. In this series, 14 airway complications occurred; 3 were dehiscence, and 11 were stenoses. No patient died as a direct result of airway complication. The only statistically significant risk factor for bronchial complication was a telescoping bronchial anastomosis. Donor ischemic time approached, but did not reach, statistical significance. All stenoses were successfully treated endoscopically, with dilatation or silastic stents as necessary, with acceptable results. These results are similar to the incidence and outcome of airway complications noted in adults. It is therefore apparent that, even in very small infants, airway complications are no higher than in adult lung transplant patients. To date, there do not appear to be any problems with long-term growth and development of the airways.

We have preferentially used absorbable suture for airway anastomoses in children in hopes that the use of such suture will not impede growth of the airway anastomosis. At moderate follow-up, there does not appear to be any evidence of progressive stricture of airways, even in very small children.

Trimming of the donor lungs as close to the right upper lobe pulmonary artery as possible, so that vascularization can occur retrograde from the transplanted lung, and use of the bilateral sequential transplant technique are associated with low rates of bronchial complications. We have used running suture technique for the membranous portion of the bronchus and interrupted suture technique for the cartilaginous portion. If size discrepancies are present, the magnitude of telescoping of the anastomosis is as minimal as possible; the smaller airway is placed inside the larger airway as necessary. Early in our experience with lung transplantation, we used omental pedicles for bronchial wraps or pericardial pedicles to protect the bronchial anastomosis from the anteriorly located pulmonary artery. During the past 4 years, however, we have not used any bronchial wrap. We loosely tack adventitial tissue in the region of the airway over the anastomoses, if it is readily available, but otherwise use no protective coverage of the bronchial anastomosis. To date, there has been no increase in airway complications with the use of this modified technique. In fact, we believe that "protecting the airway" with additional material may impede the development of new blood supply to the airway.

The issue of transplantation of the lungs with additional cardiac repair has been addressed elsewhere.[4, 5] The cardiac repair can generally be performed after removal of the recipient lungs during cardiopulmonary bypass. The heart can then reperfuse during the entire time of lung implantation in most cases, thereby resulting in the best return of cardiac function before weaning from cardiopulmonary bypass.

A unique subgroup of children includes those who have pulmonary vein stenosis. These patients often have had stents implanted in the pulmonary veins or have had multiple previous surgeries. In most of these patients, it is a minor issue to excise the pulmonary venous confluence during cardioplegic arrest at the time of lung implantation and to suture the pulmonary vein confluence of the donor lungs to the left atrium directly. On occasion, it may be necessary to implant both lungs during a single period of cardiac arrest with cardioplegia. Because both lungs have generally been removed before cross-clamping and cardioplegic arrest, the entire ischemic time on the heart for implantation of both lungs is typically less than 45 minutes. These patients have done quite well after transplant, because they have intrinsically normal cardiac function.

We have used aprotinin during lung implantation in children to decrease the bleeding from collaterals in the chest and from adhesions. Nevertheless, patients who have cyanosis and multiple collateral vessels to the lung are at significant risk for development of hemorrhage after surgery. These patients are the most difficult subgroup to treat with lung implantation. Although the presence of collaterals may not be an absolute contraindication to transplantation, they certainly increase the risk of the operative procedure. In our series, collaterals have been associated with hemorrhagic complications and death.

RESULTS

All patients who underwent transplantation in Philadelphia were in New York Heart Association class IV before the procedure; half were mechanically ventilated, and one was supported by ECMO. Among the 13 current survivors, all but one can engage in all age-appropriate activities, and all have achieved significant age-appropriate developmental milestones. One infant, who was intubated, ventilated, and treated with continuous neuromuscular blockade and sedation for 3 months before transplantation, has moderate developmental delay at 1 year of age (sits independently but does not stand; babbles but has no words) and has feeding difficulties (intermittently depends on gastrostomy feedings). All who are old enough to attend school have been able to return to full-time, regular classes 3 months after their transplant. No patient has had any airway anastomotic complications, and growth of the airways has so far been adequate.

SUMMARY AND CONCLUSIONS

Lung transplantation can offer improved quality of life and prolonged survival to children who have end-stage cardiopulmonary disease, even in the presence of characteristics that have been considered poor prognostic indicators. At present, children who have pulmonary hypertension tend to be referred for transplantation late in the course of their disease; as a result, almost half die before organs become available. Cardiac catheterization for accurate disease staging, appropriate timing of evaluation and listing for transplantation, and referral to centers experienced in the treatment of children who have end-stage cardiovascular disease are all essential components of a process that will improve survival in such children. Our experience indicates that there may be important developmental differences in the body's response to lung transplantation; thus, protocols that are suitable for older adolescents and adults may be unsuitable for young children. An integrative approach to investigation of these issues, i.e., one in which careful clinical observation and data acquisition are combined with targeted bench research, is most likely to result in insights that will directly benefit patients.

REFERENCES

1. St. Louis International Lung Transplant Registry, St Louis, April 1995.
2. Hosenpud JD, Novick RJ, Breen TJ, et al: The registry of the International Society for Heart and Lung Transplantation: Twelfth Official Report—1995. *J Heart Lung Transplant* 14:805–815, 1995.
3. Kerem E, Reisman J, Corey M, et al: Prediction of mortality in patients with cystic fibrosis. *N Engl J Med* 326:1187–1191, 1993.
4. Spray TL, Mallory GB, Canter CE, et al: Pediatric lung transplantation: Indications, techniques, and early results. *J Thorac Cardiovasc Surg* 107:990–1000, 1994.
5. Bridges ND, Mallory GB, Huddleston CB, et al: Lung transplantation for pulmonary hypertension and congenital heart disease in children and young adults. *Ann Thorac Surg* 59:813–821, 1995.
6. Rich S, Kaufmann E, Levy PS: The effect of high doses of calcium-channel blockers on survival in primary pulmonary hypertension. *N Engl J Med* 327:76–81, 1992.
7. Barst RJ, Rubin LJ, Long WA, et al: A comparison of continuous intravenous epoprostenol (prostacyclin) with conventional therapy for primary pulmonary hypertension. *N Engl J Med* 334:296–301, 1996.
8. D'Alonzo GE, Barst RJ, Ayres SM, et al: Survival in patients with primary pulmonary hypertension: Results from a national prospective registry. *Ann Int Med* 115:343–349, 1991.
9. Sandoval J, Bauerle O, Gomez A, et al: Primary pulmonary hypertension in children: Clinical characterization and survival. *J Am Coll Cardiol* 25:466–474, 1995.
10. Clabby ML, Canter CE, Moller JH, et al: Predictors of survival and time of listing for lung transplantation in children with Eisenmenger syndrome or primary pulmonary hypertension. *Circulation* 92:1S–247S, 1995.

11. Mendeloff EN, Spray TL, Huddleston CB, et al: Lung transplantation for congenital pulmonary vein stenosis. *Ann Thorac Surg* 60:903–907, 1995.
12. Bridges ND, Gaynor JW, Spray TL: Outcome of children with pulmonary hypertension listed for lung or heart/lung transplantation, submitted.
13. Kerstein D, Levy PS, Hsu DT, et al: Blade balloon atrial septostomy in patients with severe primary pulmonary hypertension. *Circulation* 91:2028–2035, 1995.
14. Forty J, Hasan A, Gould FK, et al: Single lung transplantation with simultaneous contralateral pneumonectomy for cystic fibrosis. *J Heart Lung Transplant* 13:727–730, 1994.
15. Bridges ND, Mallory GB, Huddleston CB, et al: Lung transplantation in infancy and early childhood. *J Heart Lung Transplant,* in press.
16. Ho M, Jaffe R, Miller G, et al: The frequency of Epstein-Barr virus infection and associated lymphoproliferative syndrome after transplantation and its manifestations in children. *Transplantation* 45:719–727, 1988.
17. Huddleston CB, Spray TL, Mallory G: Airway complications following pediatric lung transplantation. *J Heart Lung Transplant,* in press.

Dynamic Cardiomyoplasty

Luiz Felipe P. Moreira , M.D., Ph.D.
Cardiovascular Surgeon, Heart Institute, São Paulo University Medical School, Brazil

Noedir A.G. Stolf, M.D., Ph.D.
Associated Professor, Department Cardio-Thoracic Surgery; Cardiovascular Surgeon, Heart Institute, São Paulo University Medical School, Brazil

Advances in the treatment of chronic heart failure must constitute a health care priority, given the increasing incidence and prevalence of the disorder and its marked effect on quality of life and life expectancy. Within the past decade, an extraordinary improvement in the pharmacologic management of heart failure was observed. The mortality rate among patients who have symptomatic cardiomyopathies remains unacceptably high, however, despite the use of optimal medical therapy.[1]

Heart transplantation is recognized as the only viable therapeutic option for patients who have end-stage heart disease, with overall 5- and 10-year survival rates of 62% and 48%, respectively.[2] Nevertheless, the shortage of donors and the increasing number of candidates who require urgent treatment have decreased the number of heart transplants for outpatient candidates.[3] This situation justifies the use of alternate surgical options for patients who have moderate or severe cardiomyopathies and cannot have a reasonable quality of life and good prognosis with medical therapy. This population currently represents more than 2,200 patients who are awaiting transplantation in the United States alone; these patients have only a 4% chance of receiving a heart each month.[3]

Dynamic cardiomyoplasty is a surgical technique that uses electrically stimulated skeletal muscles to partially replace or reinforce the heart muscle in the treatment of advanced cardiomyopathies. The primary objectives of this technique are to reverse congestive heart failure and halt the progression of the underlying disease by increasing ventricular pumping performance and reinforcing ventricular walls.

Dynamic cardiomyoplasty was introduced clinically by Carpentier and Chachques[4] in 1985. Since then, this technique has

Advances in Cardiac Surgery®, vol. 8
© 1996, Mosby–Year Book, Inc.

been cautiously evaluated worldwide and has been performed in more than 700 patients. This international experience also includes a multicenter clinical trial done with the coordination of Medtronic, Inc., which enrolled 360 patients until the last public domain report on April 1994.

In this chapter, we discuss in detail the present indications, technical aspects, general results, and perspectives of clinical cardiomyoplasty. Further, we emphasize the current benefits and limitations of the procedure as an alternative to heart transplantation in the treatment of severe cardiomyopathies.

BACKGROUND

The idea of using skeletal muscle grafts as a source of energy to support the failing heart is appealing. Skeletal muscles are better generators of contractile work than is cardiac muscle in terms of the power that can develop during a single contraction and the force that can be exerted per unit of cross-sectional area.[5] Some biological constraints need to be overcome, however, to allow their use in long-term circulatory assistance.

In 1959, Kantrowitz and McKinnon[6] were the first to apply an electrically stimulated skeletal muscle graft to augment arterial blood pressure, but the difficulty of overcoming the inherent problem of muscle fatigue caused by continuous stimulation impeded further advances at that time. Only after the discovery, in the late 1960s, that skeletal muscle can be transformed after six to eight weeks of chronic electrical stimulation to fatigue-resistant, purely type I fibers, was this constraint resolved.[5,7] The increased resistance to fatigue arises from a combination of two factors: a decrease in the energy requirements of the muscle and an enhanced capacity for generating that energy through aerobic routes. In response to chronic stimulation, a transition occurs from myosin heavy and light chain isoforms of the type II fast muscle to those characteristics of the type I slow muscle.[7]

The second constraint was represented by the small and short duration twitch observed in a single skeletal muscle contraction, which would have little effect on circulatory support. In this regard, the sequential addition of electrical pulses leads to the summation of skeletal muscle twitches, thereby increasing both the duration and the force of contraction.[8] Consequently, the clinical application of dynamic cardiomyoplasty was possible after the development of implantable pulse generators that could deliver pulse train stimulation.

INDICATION CRITERIA

Dynamic cardiomyoplasty has been performed in the treatment of patients who have dilated or ischemic cardiomyopathies. The international experience also includes patients who underwent this procedure for treatment of Chagas' disease cardiomyopathy and left ventricular tumor or aneurysm (Fig 1). The preoperative demographics of patients who underwent surgery as part of the Medtronic multicenter study[9] shows a similar distribution of heart failure etiologies (dilated cardiomyopathy, 51%; ischemic cardiomyopathy, 46%; other, 3%). On the other hand, 85.7% of the 112 patients who underwent surgery in South American centers until October 1994[10] had the diagnosis of dilated cardiomyopathy; this higher percentage was also observed among the 41 patients in the São Paulo University Heart Institute series.

In general, dynamic cardiomyoplasty is indicated for patients who have a high risk of dying of severe cardiomyopathies; this indication does not essentially differ from heart transplantation criteria.[11] Candidates for this procedure are normally screened on the basis of factors that have been related to mortality in patients who have congestive heart failure. These factors include the existence of significant functional limitation despite attempts to optimize medical therapy with maximal doses of diuretics and angiotensin-converting enzyme inhibitors, as defined by the presence of New

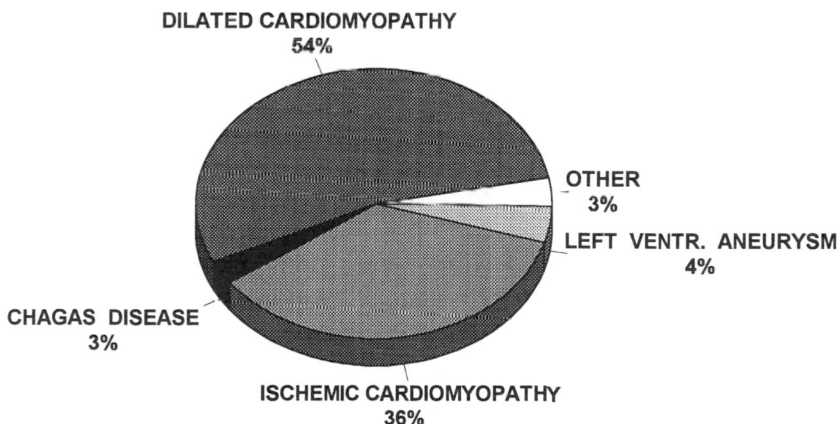

FIGURE 1.

Indications of dynamic cardiomyoplasty in the international experience. Data on 458 patients who underwent surgery from January 1985 to May 1994.

York Heart Association (NYHA) class III or IV symptoms, recurrent hospitalizations for congestive heart failure, or peak oxygen consumption during exercise testing of less than 16 mL/kg/min. Other factors used to define indication for cardiomyoplasty are indexes relating to cardiac pump dysfunction, such as left ventricular ejection fraction of less than 25%, cardiac output of less than 2.5 L/min/m^2 at rest, and high left ventricular filling pressures (pulmonary wedge pressure or left ventricular end-diastolic pressure of more than 15 mm Hg).

Patients who undergo dynamic cardiomyoplasty need to be stable enough with medical therapy to withstand a waiting period of two to three months before effective adaptation of the skeletal muscle flap. Patients who are receiving intravenous (IV) inotropic drugs, therefore, are not candidates for cardiomyoplasty. Persistent functional class IV has also been defined as a contraindication to this procedure.[9, 10] Other factors considered contraindications to cardiomyoplasty are the existence of important or severe valvular dysfunction; arrhythmias not controlled by medical therapy; major enlargement of the left ventricle, with internal diastolic diameter of more than 5 cm/m^2; diagnosis of hypertrophic cardiomyopathy, with systemic diastolic blood pressure of more than 95 mm Hg; poor lung function, with forced vital capacity of less than 55% of predicted value; unresolved drug or alcohol abuse; and any life-threatening noncardiac disease. In addition, patients who have important pulmonary hypertension, chronic atrial fibrillation, or peak oxygen consumption of less than 10 mL/kg/min have shown poor long-term outcome with this procedure, as we discuss in the Results section of this chapter.

TECHNICAL CONSIDERATIONS

SURGICAL PROCEDURE

Skeletal Muscle Flap Dissection and Transposition

The left latissimus dorsi muscle has been used most frequently for dynamic cardiomyoplasty, because of its anatomical proximity to the heart, its large bulk, and its predominant axial neurovascular pedicle, which is suitable for electrode placement and stimulation.[8] In addition, the use of this muscle as a graft causes negligible functional impairment for the patient. Other muscles may be also used. For example, the right latissimus dorsi has been used for selected patients, particularly those who have ischemic cardiomyopathy without an important left ventricular enlargement.[12]

Dynamic cardiomyoplasty is usually performed through two separated incisions: a lateral approach for muscle flap dissection and a subsequent medium sternotomy for cardiac access.[8, 13] This operation can also be done with a single lateral incision in the left hemithorax when it is performed as an isolated procedure. The advantage of using a single incision, however, is offset by the limited exposure of the heart and the high incidence of wound infection.[8]

For dissection of the latissimus dorsi muscle,[8, 13] a longitudinal incision from the axilla toward the posterior iliac crest is normally made. The muscle graft is separated from surrounding tissues and from its distal insertions, thereby preserving the superior neurovascular pedicle. Two intramuscular (IM) pacing electrodes are implanted for muscle flap stimulation. The cathode is positioned near the course of the main nerve branches, and the anode is placed 5 or 7 cm distal to the cathode. Electrophysiologic tests for threshold and impedance are performed, but without the use of curariform drugs. The latissimus dorsi muscle and the implanted electrodes are then transposed into the left hemithorax through a window created by partial resection of the anterior portion of the second or third rib.

Wrapping Procedure

The fixation of the latissimus dorsi muscle around the ventricular walls is normally performed without cardiopulmonary bypass, which has been used only when dynamic cardiomyoplasty is associated with other procedures. The muscle graft may be fixed directly to the myocardium or to the pericardium by separated sutures. With the first approach,[13, 14] four or five sutures are placed in the left ventricle along the posterior atrioventricular line and, after fixation of the muscle flap, behind the heart; additional sutures are placed in the diaphragmatic and anterior walls of the right ventricle. In the noncardiac suture technique,[8] two stay sutures are placed to align the edge of the muscle flap to the posterior atrioventricular groove of the left ventricle; one is placed at the posterior pericardium near the left atrium appendage, and the other is placed in the pericardium near the junction of the inferior vena cava and right atrium. The remainder of the muscle is turned around the apex and approximated to the anterior and lateral borders of the heart by interrupted sutures.

The muscle fibers are normally oriented to wrap the heart in a clockwise fashion as viewed from the apex; either the costal[14] or the subcutaneous surface[8] of the latissimus dorsi muscle faces the epicardium (Fig 2). These approaches allow the left latissimus

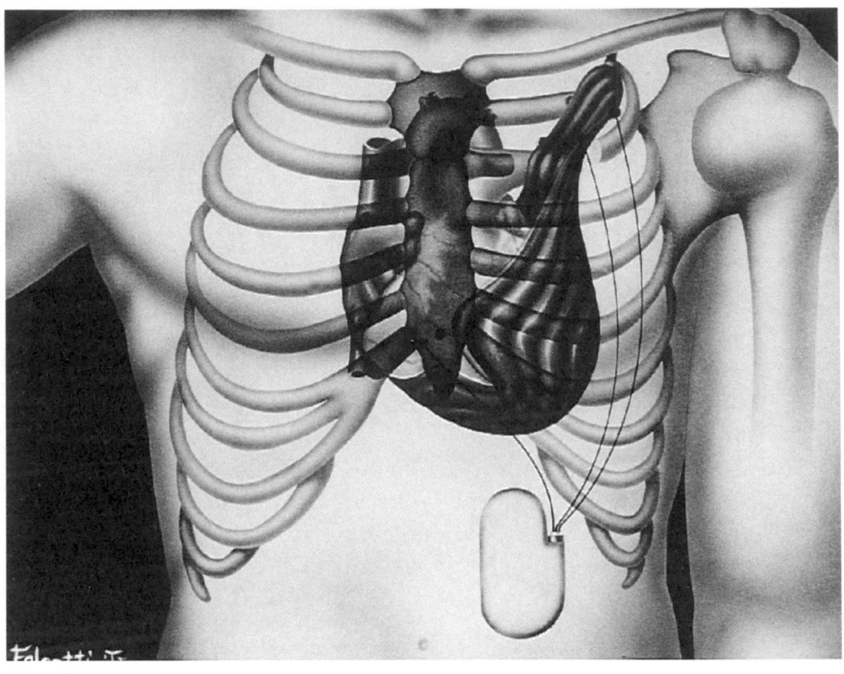

FIGURE 2.
Schematic representation of dynamic cardiomyoplasty using the left latissiimus dorsi muscle wrapped around the ventricular walls with its costal surface facing the epicardium.

dorsi muscle to cover the left ventricular free wall almost completely. In many patients who have large hearts, however, the right ventricular free wall cannot be fully covered by the muscle graft; the use of autologous or bovine pericardium patches is then necessary to complete the wrap.

Before the closure of the chest cavity, an epimyocardial sensing lead is placed in either the left or the right ventricle. Finally, an abdominal subcutaneous or submuscular pocket is fashioned, and the electrodes are tunneled to the pocket and connected to the cardiomyostimulator.

Anesthetic management

Specific aspects of the anesthetic management of patients undergoing dynamic cardiomyoplasty must be emphasized, because this operation is normally performed in patients at high risk and the mean anesthesia time ranges from six to ten hours. The systematic use of dopamine, dobutamine, and sodium nitroprusside, associated with the maintenance of adequate volume loading, is often necessary to improve the hemodynamic profile and to allow the stability of arterial blood pressure, especially during the muscle heart wrapping procedure.[15] The prophylactic use of IV inotropic support is normally maintained at least one week after the operation.

Monitoring of neuromuscular blockade is important to avoid interference with electrophysiologic testing of the muscle flap. Further, a double-lumen endobronchial tube has been used to perform one-lung ventilation during resection of the ribs and introduction of the muscle flap into the thoracic cavity.[15] Finally, the placement of an epidural catheter has also been proposed to help with pulmonary care during the first days after surgery.

SKELETAL MUSCLE FLAP STIMULATION

Synchronizable burst stimulators have been frequently used in the dynamic cardiomyoplasty clinical experience.[8–10] The use of single-pulse cardiac pacemakers for muscle flap stimulation was also reported, however, in some clinical series.[16, 17] In both cases, the muscle flap is stimulated to contract in synchronism with the heart, triggered by the R wave of the ECG.

Skeletal muscle flap stimulation normally starts only two weeks after cardiomyoplasty, and a progressive muscle conditioning protocol is followed for an additional six to eight weeks.[8] The interval between the surgical procedure and the beginning of muscle flap stimulation allows the distal part of the muscle to recover from the loss of its blood supply and allows adhesions to develop between the flap and the ventricular epicardium.

During the late postoperative period, the skeletal muscle flap may be synchronized to every other cardiac beat, or in 1:1 mode with the heart rate.[8] Pulse train stimulation is normally used with a burst frequency of 30 Hz and is associated with supramaximal pulse amplitude values to avoid ineffective muscle flap contraction. The delay between the ventricular-sensed event and the muscle burst needs to be adjusted with the use of echocardiographic monitoring to provide an exact synchronization between the muscle flap contraction and ventricular systole (Fig 3). Several authors have positioned the beginning of the muscle burst immediately after the closure of the mitral valve.[8, 14] Recent reports, however, have discussed the importance of the individual tuning of the synchronization interval based on aortic flow measurements to provide better ventricular assistance.[18, 19]

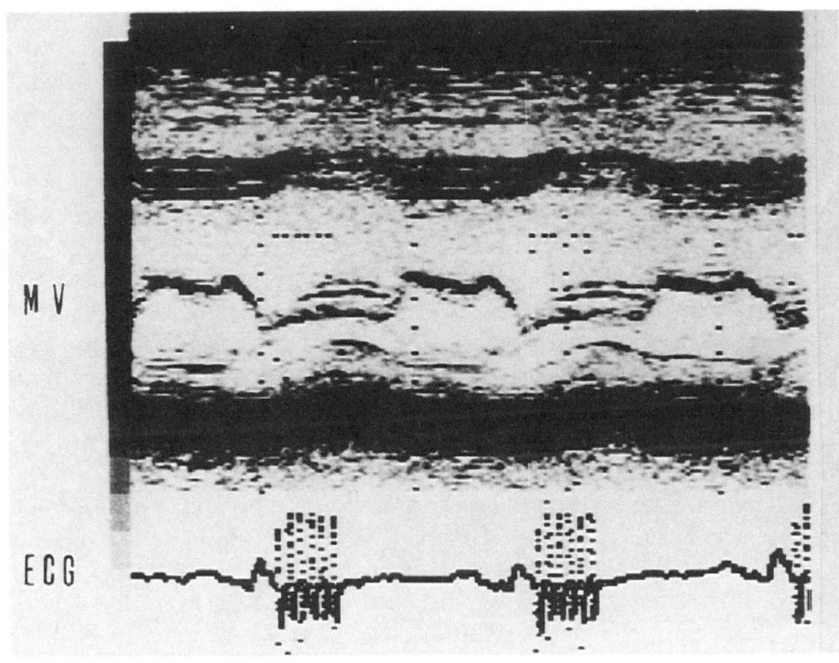

FIGURE 3.
M-mode echocardiogram showing the synchronization between muscle flap contraction and ventricular systole, with the muscle burst adjusted to start immediately after the closure of the mitral valve. (Courtesy of Jatene AD, Moreira LFP, Stolf NAG, et al: Left ventricular function changes after cardiomyoplasty in patients with dilated cardiomyopathy. *J Thorac Cardiovasc Surg* 102:133, 1991.)

RESULTS

IMMEDIATE SURGICAL RESULTS

Hospital mortality rates after dynamic cardiomyoplasty have varied in the largest clinical series from 0% to 23%.[20–24] The Medtronic worldwide experience presented an overall mortality rate of 18% and showed that procedure-related deaths occurred in 16 of 45 patients (36%) who were in functional class IV and in 43 of 272 patients (16%) in NYHA class III. Further, the overall hospital mortality rate in this trial decreased to less than 10% among patients who entered the study after a center had performed its first ten procedures. By contrast, the 30-day mortality rate after cardiomyoplasty in the overall experience of South American centers was only 8.1%.[10] The absence of patients who underwent associated procedures and the absence of cardiopulmonary bypass in this series may explain the differences.

The reasons for immediate postoperative deaths are mainly related to primary ventricular failure.[9, 10, 20, 21, 24] Arrhythmia-related deaths have also been reported in most clinical series.[9, 10, 20, 21] Surgical factors that have been correlated to operative mortality include the use of cardiopulmonary bypass and the requirement for an intra-aortic balloon pump at the time of the operation.[25] Preoperative functional class IV and poor right ventricular ejection fraction were also significantly correlated with operative mortality in some clinical series.[9, 25, 26]

Another important aspect related to the immediate postoperative period is the possibility of skeletal muscle flap ischemic compromise after the cardiomyoplasty procedure.[24, 27] This complication may lead to the absence of muscle flap contraction with electrical stimulation, which could compromise the clinical and left ventricular function benefits of the operation. There is no reliable method to detect this complication early, but its appearance may be suggested by important increases in levels of creatinokynase enzymes immediately after surgery.[27]

MECHANISMS OF ACTION

Influence on Left Ventricular Function

Several mechanisms seem to account for the improvement observed in ventricular function after dynamic cardiomyoplasty. In addition to the enhancement of left ventricular systolic function by the direct action of synchronized skeletal muscle flap contraction, several studies have suggested that cardiomyoplasty may work like an elastic girdle around the heart, helping to reverse chamber remodeling. Moreover, both mechanisms may ultimately be responsible for improved diastolic function properties and for the decrease of ventricular wall stress, which may subsequently contribute to improved myocardial oxygen balance. These concepts are summarized in Figure 4 and are discussed in detail below.

The improvement of left ventricular systolic function has been consistently reported in most clinical series. Several authors documented that radioisotopic left ventricular ejection fraction increases approximately 15% to 40% in relation to preoperative data, 6 months after dynamic cardiomyoplasty.[12, 17, 25, 27] This finding was also demonstrated by the Medtronic multicenter clinical trial, which showed a significant improvement of this parameter from 21.3 ± 6.8% to 24.6 ± 9.5%. In addition to these findings, a more significant change in left ventricular ejection fraction has been demonstrated after cardiomyoplasty by heart catheterization. Carpentier and colleagues[25] documented that this variable increased from 24% to 30.6% in 20 patients whose status was followed more than two years. Jegaden et al.[28] reported similar results in six patients who underwent two years of follow-up. In the São Paulo Heart Institute series,[29] left ventricular regional wall motion was analyzed in ten patients before and 16 months after the operation; the findings indicated that the significant improvement in ejection fraction (from 15.1 ± 7.9% to 30.9 ± 8.3%) resulted from similar modifications of anterobasal, anterolateral, apical, diaphragmatic, and posterobasal regions (Fig 5). Also important is the fact that this study demonstrated the decrease of left ventricular ejection fraction to 23.1 ± 13.4% when the myostimulator was turned off for 24 hours, which ruled out the possibility of a placebo effect.

Regarding other hemodynamic parameters, the Medtronic multicenter study also documented the significant improvement of stroke volume index (from 29.3 ± 8.2 to 32.3 ± 10.6 mL/m^2) after dynamic cardiomyoplasty. Several authors reported similar results, but these studies failed to demonstrate significant changes in the

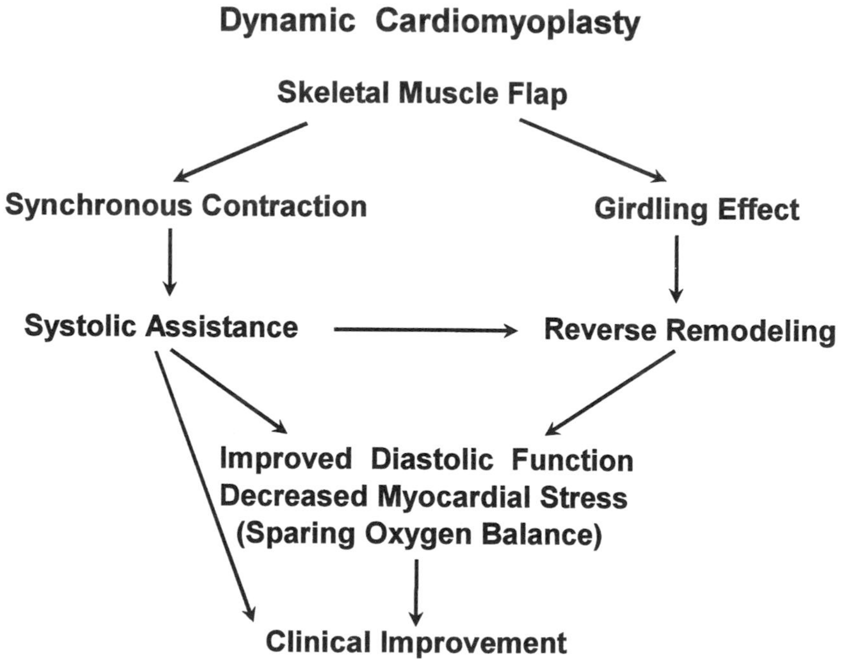

FIGURE 4.
Schematic representation of dynamic cardiomyoplasty mechanisms of action.

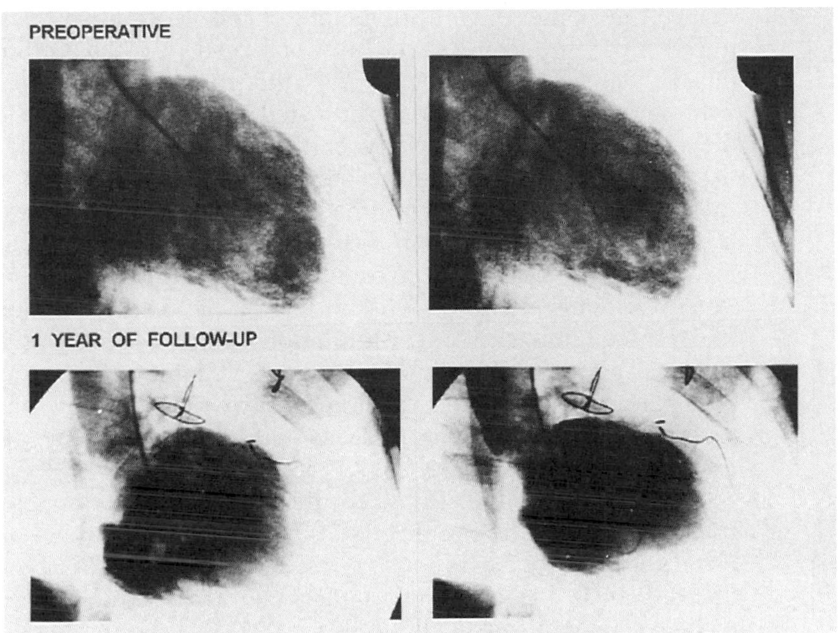

FIGURE 5.

Left ventricular angiography in diastole and systole at the preoperative period and at one year of follow-up, showing the improvement of ejection fraction and the decrease of end-diastolic and end-systolic volumes after dynamic cardiomyoplasty. (Courtesy of Moreira LFP, Bocchi EA, Bacal F, et al: Present trends in clinical experience with dynamic cardiomyoplasty. *Artif Organs* 19:213, 1995, published by International Society of Artificial Internal Organs, Cleveland, Ohio.)

pulmonary pressures or in other hemodynamic parameters in the cardiomyoplasty follow-up.[12, 22, 25, 28] In addition to the significant increase of stroke volume index (from 20.2 ± 3 to 24.9 ± 7.2 mL/m^2) observed during 6 months of follow-up in São Paulo study,[14, 27] significant improvement of left ventricular stroke work index (from 17.5 ± 5.2 to 25.5 ± 9.1 g-m/m^2) was documented after cardiomyoplasty. This improvement was associated with a significant decrease of pulmonary pressures. More evident changes in cardiac output and global circulatory function were also documented at peak of a treadmill exercise test in three of these patients.[30]

Other reports have demonstrated the direct influence of skeletal muscle flap contraction on left ventricular systolic function by comparing the results obtained under stimulated and nonstimulated beats or with the myostimulator turned on and off. In addition to the significant improvement of left ventricular stroke volume, on the order of 20% to 30% observed in these studies with muscle flap stimulation,[22, 25, 28, 31] the analysis of the pressure-volume relationship has also indicated a better contractile state of the combined ventricular myocardium and wrapped latissimus dorsi muscle. Schreuder et al.[31] documented the leftward shift of the end-systolic pressure-volume points, the increase of peak ejection rate, and the increase of peak negative dP/dt when the applied myostimulator settings are tuned to the patients' best settings. Moreover, Bellotti and co-workers[32] from São Paulo demonstrated that skeletal muscle flap stimulation increased left ventricular maximal elastance (from 17 ± 1 to 21 ± 1 mm Hg/cm) in eight patients who had dilated cardiomyopathy. This finding was associated with the significant decrease of left ventricular end-diastolic pressure (from 27.1 ± 2.8 to 17.6 ± 1.7 mm Hg).

As first reported in animal studies, the improvement of left ventricular systolic function through the action of an external impulse unrelated to the cardiac muscle itself may also decrease ventricular wall stress[33] and lead to a consequent reduction in myocardial oxygen consumption.[34] This finding was clinically documented in the São Paulo study[32] with the use of pressure-volume loops obtained with the myostimulator turned on and off for 24 hours. Significant reduction of left ventricular end-systolic stress, from 175 ± 12 to 149 ± 10 g/cm^2, and of left ventricular end-diastolic stress, from 69 ± 8 to 37 ± 5 g/cm^2, were demonstrated by data obtained with the myostimulator turned on and turned off. With regard to diastolic function, this study further demonstrated that left ventricular chamber stiffness was significantly decreased by approximately 56% and that left ventricular filling was also influenced by cardiomyoplasty. Alterations in left ventricular diastolic, rather than systolic, function were also reported by Jondeau and coworkers[35] with skeletal muscle flap assistance. In that study, a significant decrease of Doppler E/A waves ratio was documented after stimulation of latissimus dorsi muscle was discontinued in ten patients evaluated at least 6 months after the operation.

In addition to the direct influence of muscle flap contraction on left ventricular function, experimental reports have also postulated that dynamic cardiomyoplasty may work as an active or even passive support of the damaged myocardium.[36–38] The muscle wrap may provide an elastic constraint to the ventricular walls, thereby limiting cardiac dilatation much like a girdle. Reverse remodeling or prevention of further ventricular dilatation are the possible consequences of these mechanisms. Kass et al.[39] performed serial pressure-volume studies in three patients who had dilated cardiomyopathy and suggested that cardiomyoplasty benefits were derived less from the active systolic assistance than from remodeling, perhaps because of an external elastic constraint. The experimental study of Capouya and co-workers[36] also supports this concept. These authors demonstrated that hearts previously wrapped with a nonstimulated skeletal muscle graft had less chamber enlargement and less decline in ejection fraction than did those without previous cardiomyoplasty in a model of progressive heart failure induced by rapid pacing.

The reverse remodeling after dynamic cardiomyoplasty is finally indicated by the observation that improvement in left ventricular function is normally associated with a decrease in left ventricular end-diastolic volume and pressure. This fact was primarily documented by Bocchi and co-workers[29] from São Paulo, who showed that the left ventricle became markedly more spheric in the diastole and with a decreased major-to-minor axis ratio in the studies performed during the postoperative period (Fig 5). Changes in the process of ventricular dilatation were also suggested by data obtained from pressure-volume studies in both experimental[37] and clinical investigations.[38]

The effect of left ventricular chamber reverse remodeling would explain why patients experience significant symptomatic improvement with muscle flap stimulation in a 1:6 or 1:8 ratio with the heart rate.[40] This improvement is also seen when the procedure is performed only with single pulses, as in some clinical series.[16, 17] Finally, another mechanism that may influence the outcome of dynamic cardiomyoplasty in patients who have ischemic cardiomyopathy is the possibility of cross-revascularization between the muscle flap and the ventricular epicardium, as demonstrated in the experimental studies of Beyer et al.[41] and Bailey et al.[42] and in the clinical experience of Akhmedov and colleagues[43] from Tomsk.

Several authors have discussed the importance of ventricular remodeling, defined as a change in chamber volume and shape not related to a preload-mediated increase in sarcomere length, for the syndrome of heart failure.[44] Further, the increases in ventricular wall stress and myocardial oxygen consumption observed with the remodeling process have been identified as being among the principal mechanisms in the progression of heart failure in patients who have severe cardiomyopathies.[45] In a dilated, failing left ventricle, therefore, some of the primary pathophysiologic abnormalities seem to be partially corrected after dynamic cardiomyoplasty, and slow progression of the underlying disease could result from these modifications. That this may have occurred is indicated by the maintenance of improvement in left ventricular function for up to five years after cardiomyoplasty in the São Paulo Heart Institute series (Table 1).[46] Further, data from the largest single-unit series at Broussais Hospital in Paris[25] show the stabilization of the cardiothoracic ratio and the improvement in left ventricular ejection fraction of patients who underwent cardiomyoplasty and were seen for more than three years of follow-up.

Influence on Arrhythmias Incidence

Despite significant changes observed in left ventricular function after dynamic cardiomyoplasty, the persistence of atrial and ventricular arrhythmias in the postoperative period represents an important limitation for long-term outcome. In the São Paulo experience,[47] the number of atrial fibrillation, premature ventricular contractions, and nonsustained ventricular tachycardia episodes remained approximately the same as that observed before the operation during four years of follow-up. In this regard, ventricular arrhythmias are frequently observed in patients who have dilated cardiomyopathy, but the severity of the arrhythmias has not been consistently related to the degree of impairment in left ventricular function.[48]

CLINICAL FOLLOW-UP

Influence on Quality of Life

Clinical improvement after dynamic cardiomyoplasty has been reported as a prevailing and significant outcome in nearly all series. Patients in functional class III or IV who undergo surgery normally return to class I or II and use fewer drugs than they did before surgery. The most comprehensive data available come from the Medtronic multicenter trial and show that six months after the operation only 18% of the surviving patients remained in the same functional class, 47% had improved by one class, and 32% had improved by two or more classes. Carpentier et al.[25] also reported a significant decrease in hospitalizations per patient per year from 2.4 to 0.4 after cardiomyoplasty; the same trend was observed in the São Paulo Heart Institute series.[46]

More positive data on clinical improvement have been obtained by detailed assessment of quality of life in a subset of clinical centers in the Medtronic study. Significant improvement (changes of more than 20% from preoperative status) has been observed for daily activities, social activities, quality of interaction,

TABLE 1.
Sequential Evaluation of Ventricular Function After Dynamic Cardiomyoplasty

	Preoperation (n = 28)	Follow-up: 6 mo (n = 28)	12 mo (n = 22)	24 mo (n = 11)	36 mo (n = 6)	48 mo (n = 6)	60 mo (n = 4)
Radioisotopic scintigraphy							
LVEF (%)	19.7 ± 3.3	23.9 ± 6.6*	23.3 ± 6.5*	23.3 ± 6.2	22.5 ± 3.6	20.8 ± 3	20.5 ± 3.6
RVEF (%)	25.8 ± 7.7	24.9 ± 8.6	26.5 ± 8.[illegible]*	27.5 ± 7.3*	26.5 ± 5.4	26.2 ± 4.4	25.5 ± 5.7
Hemodynamic data							
MRAP (mm Hg)	9 ± 3.6	9.1 ± 5.3	8.9 ± 5.[illegible]	9.1 ± 6.3	6.7 ± 5.6	7.2 ± 5.6	8 ± 4.7
MPAP (mm Hg)	36.1 ± 11.2	29.8 ± 9.6*	30.3 ± 9.4*	29.8 ± 1[illegible].1*	24 ± 6.8	28.2 ± 8.4	30.5 ± 7.5
MPWP (mm Hg)	24.7 ± 6.3	18.5 ± 6*	18.2 ± 5.8*	17.9 ± 7.7*	15.2 ± 3.2*	15.5 ± 6.1	19 ± 6.6
CI (L/min/m^2)	1.94 ± 0.31	2.02 ± 0.4	2.04 ± 0.44	1.97 ± 0.26	2.3 ± 0.3	2.17 ± 0.26	2.18 ± 0.2
SI (mL/m^2)	20.6 ± 3.1	24 ± 5.3*	24.7 ± 6.8*	25 ± 6.7*	28.9 ± 4.4*	27 ± 6.8	25.7 ± 4.9
LVSW I (g-m/m^2)	17.5 ± 5.2	25.5 ± 9.1*	25.6 ± 9.4*	25.4 ± 7*	30.9 ± 9.5*	29.7 ± 10.9*	25.5 ± 8.5

Abbreviations: LVEF, left ventricular ejection fraction; *RVEF,* right ventricular ejection fraction; *MRAP,* mean right atrium pressure; *MPAP,* mean pulmonary artery pressure; *MPWP,* mean pulmonary wedge pressure; *MAP,* mean arterial pressure; *CI,* cardiac index; *SI,* systolic index; *LVSW I,* left ventricular stroke work index.

*$p < 0.05$ in relation to preoperative data of matched patients.

(Adapted from Moreira LFP, Stolf NAG, Bocchi EA, et al: Clinical and left ventricular function outcomes up to five years after dynamic cardiomyoplasty. *J Thorac Cardiovasc Surg* 109:353–363, 1995.)

and mental health in more than 70% of the surviving patients. Similar results are reported by Borghetti-Maio and co-workers from São Paulo.[49] These authors also suggest that cardiomyoplasty significantly reduces the degree of limitation for physical activities, sleep pattern, food pattern, and perceptions and expectations about the treatment.

When evaluating exercise capacity, however, analysis of the Medtronic multicenter data failed to demonstrate any significant change of exercise parameters after dynamic cardiomyoplasty. Otherwise, improvement in maximum oxygen consumption (peak Vo_2) and in total exercise time have been found in some single series. Carpentier and associates[25] reported a significant increase in Vo_2 on the order of 45% (from 12.8 ± 3.5 to 18.6 ± 4 mL/kg/min) in patients evaluated during more than six months of follow-up. In the last report from the São Paulo University study, Bocchi and colleagues[50] showed a trend that did not achieve statistically significant improvement in peak Vo_2 in the entire group. Nevertheless, significant improvement of this parameter (from 11.1 ± 1.9 to 16.4 ± 6.2 mL/kg/min) and of exercise time (from 585 ± 77 to 825 ± 186 seconds) were documented in patients who had a preoperative peak Vo_2 of less than 14 mL/kg/min, which suggests that cardiomyoplasty seems to improve exercise parameters, at least in selected patients who have more restricted exercise capacity.

Influence on Long-term Survival

In the dynamic cardiomyoplasty long-term follow-up, late deaths have been reported despite the improvement observed in clinical and left ventricular function after surgery. Figure 6 shows the actuarial survival after cardiomyoplasty during a five-year period according to the Medtronic multicenter database and to the experience of the South American centers.[10] Figure 6 also displays the five-year survival curve obtained in the combined analysis of the long-term results of 127 patients from three major centers of the Medtronic study: Broussais Hospital, Paris; São Paulo University Heart Institute; and St. Vincent Hospital, Portland, Oregon.[51] This subset experience corresponds to one third the total Medtronic study population. From these curves, the overall one-year survival rate for dynamic cardiomyoplasty ranges from 72% to 78%. The two-year survival rate is 57% to 60%. Thereafter, there is approximately a 5.5% mortality rate per year during the subsequent years.

The causes for long-term mortality after dynamic cardiomyoplasty can be equally divided between primary ventricular failure and arrhythmia deaths in all clinical series. Primary ventricular failure occurs mainly in patients who have more important preoperative compromise and in those who had complications of the underlying disease[10, 20, 21, 24] or evidence of skeletal muscle flap ischemia immediately after surgery.[27] Otherwise, the incidence of sudden cardiac death has been less important than that described in the literature of approximately 20% to 30% per year in patients who have chronic heart failure.[52] This event, however, can be viewed as an interaction among structural abnormalities of the heart, transient functional disturbances, and the specific electrophysiologic events responsible for fatal arrhythmias. The causes are therefore multifactorial, and the relative value of each factor is unknown, which makes the incidence of this complication probably not affected by cardiomyoplasty. Bocchi et al.[47] documented that sudden cardiac death may occur during follow-up in inclusive patients who have important improvement in clinical and left ventricular function after the operation.

It is important to emphasize that the current indications for dynamic cardiomyoplasty include mainly patients at high risk of dying within one year. Accordingly, the São Paulo Heart Institute[53] reported that the survival rate among patients who underwent car-

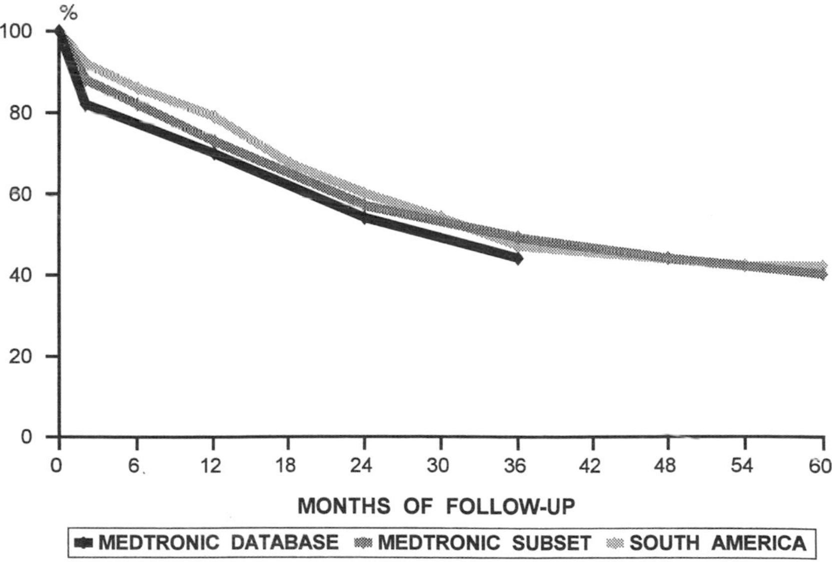

FIGURE 6.

Actuarial survival curves after dynamic cardiomyoplasty during a 5-year period according to the Medtronic multicenter database, Medtronic subset analysis,[51] and South American centers experience.[10]

diomyoplasty was much more favorable than the survival rate of a comparable, but not randomized, group of patients who received medical therapy. In that study, patients who underwent cardiomyoplasty had a survival rate of 65% at two years of follow-up, whereas the two-year survival rate was only 27% in the medically treated group. The absence, however, of randomized clinical trials to compare outcomes between cardiomyoplasty and medical therapy precludes definitive conclusions regarding the effect of this surgical procedure on long-term survival of patients who have advanced heart failure.

Factors Affecting Long-term Outcome

Analyses of preoperative factors that adversely affect long-term survival after dynamic cardiomyoplasty have been done in single-center[24–26] and multicenter studies.[9, 10, 51] In addition to the influence of other factors on long-term outcome of cardiomyoplasty, there is a consensus that the late mortality rate after this procedure has been significantly higher among patients in functional class IV, as observed in the survival curves reported by the Medtronic multicenter trial (Fig 7) and other studies.[10, 24, 51]

Table 2 shows additional risk factors that also seems to have a statistically significant effect on the five-year mortality rate after dynamic cardiomyoplasty. They include the Chagas' disease etiology and several factors related specifically to the severity of the patient's preoperative condition.[10, 51] As observed in South American experience,[10] Chagas' disease cardiomyopathy was associated with a poor long-term survival after cardiomyoplasty, with one- and five-year survival rates of 40% and 9.5%, respectively. Chagas' disease is responsible for a high incidence of atrial and ventricular arrhythmias and for a persistent chronic active myocarditis.

On the other hand, the limited long-term survival associated with cardiomyoplasty among patients who had severe preoperative compromise of the exercise performance[51] or those who had important impairment in cardiac function[10, 51] demonstrates that this procedure should be indicated earlier than heart transplantation. In this respect, patients in the South American centers who were in functional class III or intermittent class IV and had pulmonary vascular resistance of less than four Wood units had survival rates of 82.6% at two years and 76.7% at five years of follow-up (Fig 8).[10] These values are similar to those reported after cardiac transplantation.[2] They also compare positively with recent reports of heart failure treatment in which angiotensin-converting enzyme inhibitors or vasodilators were used. These reports showed a survival

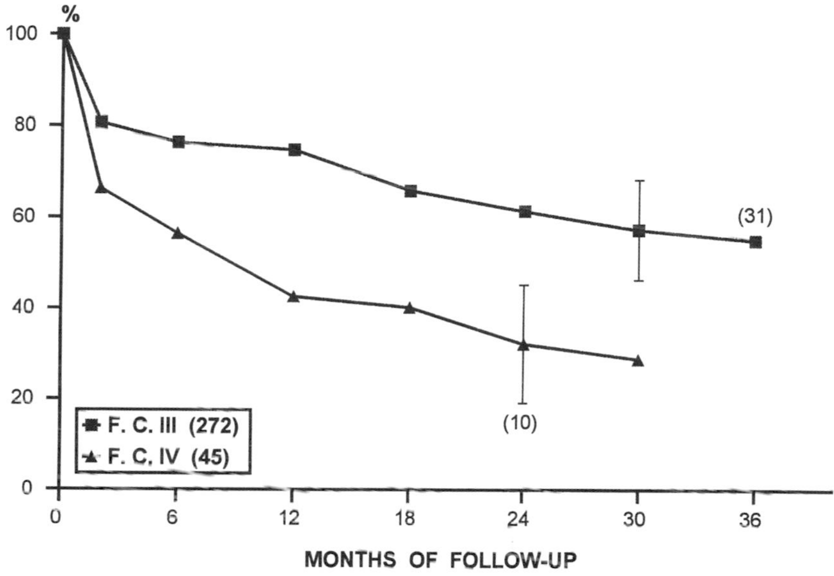

FIGURE 7.

Actuarial survival curves of patients submitted to dynamic cardiomyoplasty in New York Heart Association functional class *(FC)* III or IV, according to Medtronic multicenter study. Numbers in parenthesis indicate patients. Values are presented as mean ± 70% confidence limit.

probability of 40% to 50% in five years for patients in class III.[54, 55] Moreover, the survival expectation may be even worse with medical therapy in the presence of persistent abnormalities of hemodynamic profile,[56] as documented in most patients currently undergoing cardiomyoplasty. Finally, cardiomyoplasty does not preclude

TABLE 2.

Factors That Negatively Affect Long-term Outcome of Cardiomyoplasty*

Functional class IV
Chagas disease cardiomyopathy
Chronic atrial fibrillation
Pulmonary wedge pressure of more than 25 mm Hg
Pulmonary vascular resistance of more than 4 Wood units
Peak oxygen consumption of less than 10 mL/kg/min

*According to the Medtronic subset analysis[51] and the South American Centers experience.[10]

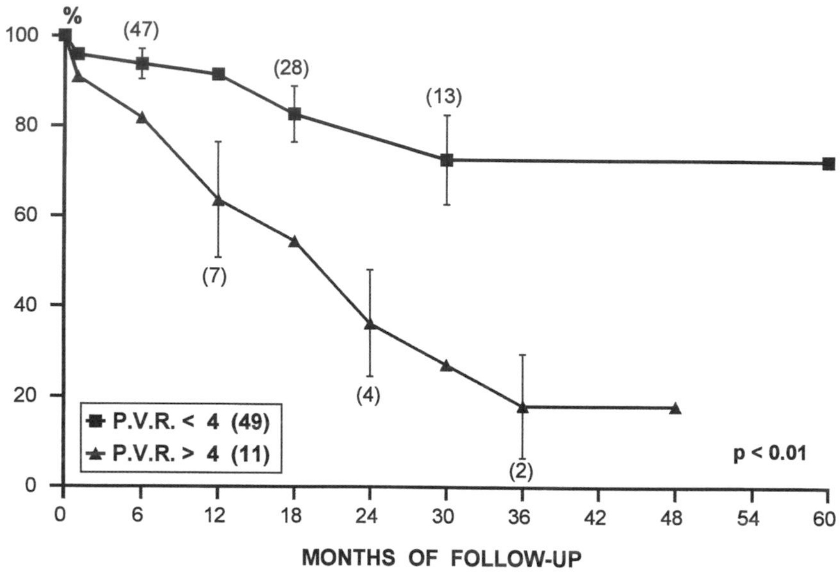

FIGURE 8.

Actuarial survival curves of patients submitted to dynamic cardiomyoplasty with preoperative pulmonary vascular resistance *(PVR)* below or above 4 Wood units, according to the experience of South American centers. Numbers in parenthesis indicate patients. Values are presented as mean ± 70% confidence limit. (Courtesy of Moreira LFP, Stolf NAG, Braile DM, et al: Dynamic cardiomyoplasty in South America. *Ann Thorac Surg* 61:410, 1996.)

future heart transplantation, which has been successfully performed by several authors during the immediate or late postoperative periods.[28, 24, 25]

SKELETAL MUSCLE FLAP PERFORMANCE AT LONG-TERM

In addition to the factors related to the underlying disease, the outcome of dynamic cardiomyoplasty may be also influenced by long-term skeletal muscle flap response to electrical stimulation. Controversial experimental results have been reported regarding the possibility of degenerative changes in the skeletal muscle flap structure after wrapping and subsequent continuous stimulation. Some animal studies showed that latissimus dorsi muscle flap may exhibit atrophy and replacement of fibers by fatty cells with chronic stimulation.[57, 58] Other authors, however, described the absence of skeletal muscle flap damage, even after long-term continuous stimulation at rates similar to those used in clinical cardiomyoplasty.[8]

Regarding the clinical experience, the São Paulo Heart Institute study[46] demonstrated that left ventricular ejection fraction tended to decrease at late follow-up and returned to preoperative levels at five years. Further, four of the five patients who survived more than five years in that series died suddenly or of progressive heart failure during seven years of follow-up. Evaluation with MRI, performed 24–52 months after surgery at the time of the cardiomyostimulator replacement in those patients, identified areas of signal intensity similar to those of subcutaneous fatty tissue in the proximal and distal parts of the wrapped latissimus dorsi muscle.[59] The existence of muscle fiber atrophy and important or severe fat tissue infiltration in the skeletal muscle flap was finally documented in necropsy studies (Fig 9).

It is important to emphasize that patients enrolled in early São Paulo experience underwent skeletal muscle flap stimulation synchronized to every cardiac beat.[46] Although the maximal rate of latissimus dorsi contractions was programmed to 100 beats per

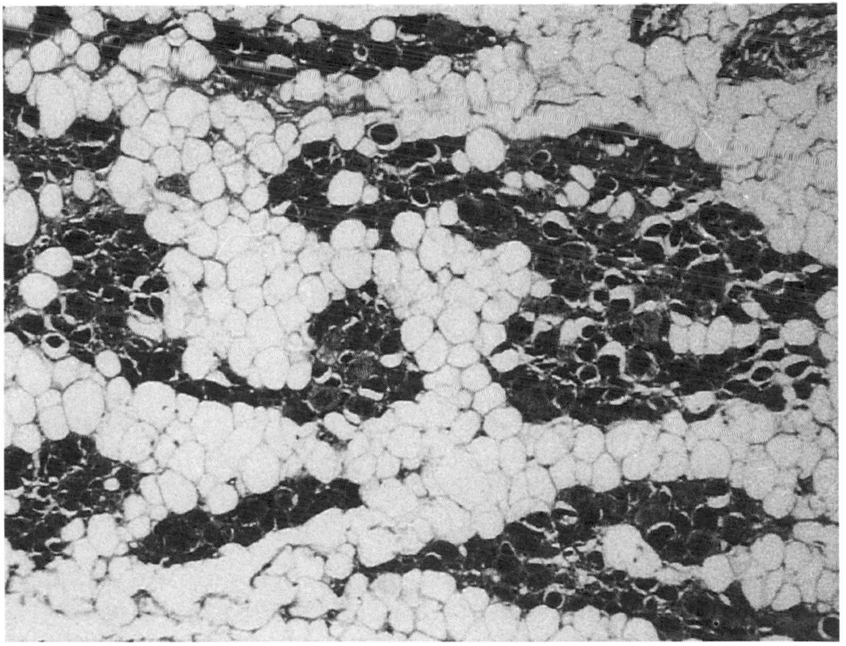

FIGURE 9.

Photomicrography of the latissimus dorsi muscle flap, obtained by necropsy study six years after dynamic cardiomyoplasty. The existence of muscle fibers atrophy and important areas of fat tissue infiltration are shown.

minute, we have since learned that this rate may be too high to allow suficient relaxation of muscle fibers with the used burst duration of 185 msec,[32, 40] thus possibly hampering muscle blood flow. This complication has not been observed in other series, including the largest clinical experience at Broussais Hospital.[21, 25] The status of these patients was maintained with muscle flap stimulation synchronized to every other cardiac beat, with the same burst duration, for more than seven years of follow-up.

Several authors have suggested that impaired muscle blood flow is the principal cause for the deterioration of latissimus dorsi muscle structure after dynamic cardiomyoplasty.[57, 58] Gealow and co-workers[60] demonstrated that skeletal muscle blood flow and force decrease when the contraction rate exceeds a specific upper rate limit for a given number of pulses in the burst. They concluded that excessive stimulation rates could be detrimental to the muscle by creating a metabolic insufficiency or ischemia. In addition the identification of the efficient working limits of conditioned skeletal muscle may be used to optimize its ability to assist cardiac function in cardiomyoplasty. With different burst stimulation patterns, e.g., a shorter duration or an adaptive feature that automatically shortens the pulse train at higher heart rates, stimulation with every heart beat may be feasible without detrimental effects, thereby potentially increasing the long-term benefits of cardiomyoplasty.

FUTURE PERSPECTIVES

The major problems limiting the success of dynamic cardiomyoplasty are related to the severity of the underlying disease, the unchanged incidence of sudden cardiac death, and the decrease of latissimus dorsi power production over time. In addition to the technological advances incorporated in the new cardiomyostimulators, which may improve long-term skeletal muscle flap performance, other developments have been discussed. A vascular delay to enhance latissimus dorsi viability immediately after surgery,[61] preoperative training protocols to increase skeletal muscle mass, and the incorporation of daily muscle flap resting periods are new approaches for improving skeletal muscle power production after the operation. Further, Fritzsche and associates[62] showed that the administration of anabolic steroids led to the acceleration of fast-to-slow twitch fibers transformation, the increase in force capacity and muscle mass of conditioned latissimus dorsi muscle, and a consequent amelioration of hemodynamic performance of cardiomyoplasty procedure.

Another technical improvement currently being evaluated is the implantation of a combined internal cardioverter-defibrillator.[63] Because of the significant incidence of sudden cardiac death among patients selected for dynamic cardiomyoplasty, this approach should dramatically reduce the long-term mortality rate, as observed among patients awaiting heart transplantation. In addition, this approach should expand the indication for cardiomyoplasty among patients who have certain arrhythmias that are not controlled by medical therapy.

The clinical application of dynamic cardiomyoplasty is limited, however, in the presence of severe left ventricular dilatation, functional incompetence of the atrioventricular valves, and important pulmonary hypertension. The possibility of left ventricular chamber reduction in patients with dilated cardiomyoplasty was recently reported by Batista et al. (unpublished data). Short-term results of reductive left ventriculoplasty, associated when necessary with mitral annuloplasty, have shown that this procedure may decrease left ventricular dimensions and volume by 25% to 40% and that this acute remodeling is normally associated with significant improvement in ejection fraction. Nevertheless, the evaluation of the hemodynamic effects of this procedure demonstrates negligible increases in stroke volume associated with the maintenance of high left ventricular filling pressures. In another study, Bolling and associates[64] reported the positive influence of the isolate correction of the secondary mitral regurgitation in end-stage cardiomyopathy. The authors suggest that mitral annuloplasty was responsible for a small but significant decrease in left ventricular end-diastolic volume and for a significant improvement in ejection fraction and stroke volume.

Accordingly, in addition to the possible effect of acute remodeling on left ventricular function, obtained either by reductive ventriculoplasty or by correction of secondary mitral regurgitation, these procedures open the possibility of a more aggressive approach for the treatment of advanced cardiomyopathies. A single-stage operation may combine the effects of these procedures to the recognized positive influence of dynamic cardiomyoplasty on left ventricular function. The first operation to combine cardiomyoplasty with reductive ventriculoplasty was performed in June 1995 at the São Paulo University Heart Institute. The procedure was named dynamic reductive ventriculomyoplasty, and the initial results have been promising. The patient had an uneventful recovery and was discharged from the hospital 10 days after surgery. Further, the reduction of left ventricular diastolic dimensions and volume allowed a better muscle flap wrapping of the ventricular surfaces. Nevertheless, to determine the appropriate place for this combined procedure in the treatment of advanced cardiomyopathies, a controlled study with a significant number of patients is needed.

REFERENCES

1. Pitt B, Cohn JN, Francis GS, et al: The effect of treatment on survival in congestive heart failure. *Clin Cardiol* 15:323–329, 1992.
2. Hosenpud JD, Novick RJ, Bree TJ, et al: The registry of the International Society for Heart and Lung Transplantation: Twelfth official report—1995. *J Heart Lung Transpl* 14:805–815, 1995.
3. Stevenson LW, Warner SL, Steimle AE, et al: The impending crisis awaiting cardiac transplantation: Modeling a solution based on selection. *Circulation* 89:450–457, 1994.
4. Carpentier A, Chachques JC: Myocardial substitution with a stimulated skeletal muscle: First successful clinical case (letter). *Lancet* 1:1267, 1985.
5. Salmons S, Jarvis JC: Cardiac assistance from skeletal muscle: A critical appraisal of the various approaches. *Br Heart J* 68:333–338, 1993.
6. Kantrowitz A, McKinnon W: The experimental use of the diaphragm as an auxiliary myocardium. *Surg Forum* 9:266–286, 1959.
7. Pette D, Vrbová G: Adaptation of mammalian skeletal muscle fibers to chronic electrical stimulation. *Rev Physiol Biochem Pharmacol* 120:115–202, 1992.
8. Carpentier A, Chachques JC, Grandjean PA: *Cardiomyoplasty.* Mount Kisco, NY, Futura, 1991.
9. Grandjean PA, Austin L, Chan S, et al: Dynamic cardiomyoplasty: Clinical follow-up results. *J Cardiac Surg* 6:80S–88S, 1991.
10. Moreira LFP, Stolf NAG, Braile DM, et al: Dynamic cardiomyoplasty in South America. *Ann Thorac Surg* 61:408–412, 1996.
11. Vagelos R, Fowler MB: Selection of patients for cardiac transplantation. *Cardiol Clin* 8:23–38, 1990.
12. Magovern JA, Park SE, Cmolik BL, et al: Early effects of right latissimus dorsi cardiomyoplasty on left ventricular function. *Circulation* 1993;88:II-298–II-303.
13. Chachques JC, Grandjean PA, Carpentier A: Latissimus dorsi cardiomyoplasty. *Ann Thorac Surg* 47:400–404, 1989.
14. Jatene AD, Moreira LFP, Stolf NAG, et al: Left ventricular function changes after cardiomyoplasty in patients with dilated cardiomyopathy. *J Thorac Cardiovasc Surg* 102:132–139, 1991.
15. Auler JOC Jr, Moreira LFP, Carvalho MJ, et al: Anesthetic management of patients undergoing cardiomyoplasty. *Anesthesiology* 77:379–381, 1992.
16. Almada H, Molteni L, Ferreira R, et al: Clinical experience with dynamic cardiomyoplasty. *J Cardiac Surg* 5:193–198, 1990.

17. García JMF, Alonso CC, Balea FD, et al: Valor de la ventriculografía isotópica en el pronóstico y seguimiento de los pacientes sometidos a miocardioplastia dinámica. *Rev Esp Cardiol* 45:381–385, 1992.
18. Grubb NR, Campanella C, Sutherland GR, et al: Optimizing muscle synchronization after dynamic cardiomyoplasty. *Eur J Cardiothorac Surg* 9:45–49, 1995.
19. Helou J, Misawa Y, Stewart JA, et al: Optimizing "delay period" for burst stimulation in dynamic cardiomyoplasty. *Ann Thorac Surg* 59:74–77, 1995.
20. Braile DM, Soares MJF, Rodrigues MCZ, et al: Cardiomyoplasty clinical study of 26 patients: A six year follow-up. *Intercont Cardiol* 2:71–78, 1993.
21. Chachques JC, Acar C, Tapia M, et al: Résultats à moyen terme de la cardiomyoplastie. *Arch Mal Coeur* 87:49–56, 1994.
22. Lorusso R, Zogno M, La Canna G, et al. Dynamic cardiomyoplasty as an effective therapy for dilated cardiomyopathy. *J Cardiac Surg* 8:177–83, 1993.
23. Magovern JA, Furnary AP, Christlieb IY, et al: Indications and risk analysis for clinical cardiomyoplasty. *Semin Thorac Cardiovasc Surg* 3:145–148, 1991.
24. Moreira LFP, Bocchi EA, Bacal F, et al: Present trends in clinical experience with dynamic cardiomyoplasty. *Artif Organs* 19:211–216, 1995.
25. Carpentier A, Chachques JC, Acar C, et al: Dynamic cardiomyoplasty at seven years. *J Thorac Cardiovasc Surg* 106:42–54, 1993.
26. Furnary AP, Magovern JA, Christlieb IY, et al: Clinical cardiomyoplasty: Preoperative factors associated with outcome. *Ann Thorac Surg* 54:1139–1143, 1992.
27. Moreira LFP, Bocchi EA, Stolf NAG, et al: Current expectations in dynamic cardiomyoplasty. *Ann Thorac Surg* 55:299–303, 1993.
28. Jegaden O, Delahaye F, Finet G, et al: Late hemodynamic results after cardiomyoplasty in congestive heart failure. *Ann Thorac Surg* 57:1151–1157, 1994.
29. Bocchi EA, Moreira LFP, Moraes AV, et al: Effects of dynamic cardiomyoplasty on regional wall motion, ejection fraction and geometry of left ventricle. *Circulation* 86:II-231–II-235, 1992.
30. Bocchi EA, Moreira LFP, Bellotti G, et al: Hemodynamic study during upright isotonic exercise before and six months after dynamic cardiomyoplasty for idiopathic dilated cardiomyopathy or Chagas' disease. *Am J Cardiol* 67:213–214, 1991.
31. Schreuder JJ, van der Veen FH, van der Velde ET, et al: Beat to beat analysis of left ventricular pressure–volume relation and stroke volume by conductance catheter and aortic modelflow in cardiomyoplasty patients. *Circulation* 91:2010–2017, 1995.
32. Bellotti G, Moraes AV, Bocchi EA, et al: Late effects of cardiomyoplasty on left ventricular mechanics and diastolic filling. *Circulation* 88:II-304–II-308, 1993.

33. Lee KF, Dignan RJ, Parmar JM, et al: Effects of dynamic cardiomyoplasty on left ventricular performance and myocardial mechanics in dilated cardiomyopathy. *J Thorac Cardiovasc Surg* 102:124–131, 1991.
34. Kawaguchi O, Goto Y, Futaki S, et al: Mechanical enhancement and myocardial oxygen saving by synchronized dynamic left ventricular compression. *J Thorac Cardiovasc Surg* 103:573–581, 1992.
35. Jondeau G, Dorent R, Bors V, et al: Dynamic cardiomyoplasty: Effect of discontinuing latissimus dorsi muscle stimulation on left ventricular systolic and diastolic performance and exercise capacity. *J Am Coll Cardiol* 26:129–134, 1995.
36. Capouya ER, Gerder RS, Drinkwater DC, et al: Girdling effect of nonstimulated cardiomyoplasty on left ventricular function. *Ann Thorac Surg* 56:867–871, 1993.
37. Cho PW, Levin HR, Curtis WE, et al: Pressure-volume analysis of changes in cardiac function in chronic cardiomyoplasty. *Ann Thorac Surg* 56:38–45, 1993.
38. Nakajima H, Niinami H, Hooper TL, et al: Cardiomyoplasty: Probable mechanism of effectiveness using the pressure-volume relationship. *Ann Thorac Surg* 57:407–415, 1994.
39. Kass DA, Baughman KL, Pak PH, et al: Reverse remodeling from cardiomyoplasty in human heart failure: External constrain versus active assist. *Circulation* 91:2314–2318, 1995.
40. Perkasky VV, Akhmedov ShD, Dubrovsky IA, et al: Optimal electrical stimulation for latissimus dorsi muscle after cardiomyoplasty. *J Cardiac Surg* 8:172–176, 1993.
41. Beyer M, Hoffer H, Eggeling T, et al: Cardiomyoplasty to improve myocardial collateral blood supply as an alternative to transplantation in intractable angina. *J Heart Lung Transplant* 11:189S–191S, 1992.
42. Bailey WF Jr, Magno MG, Buckman PD, et al: Chronic stimulation enhances extramyocardial collateral blood flow after a cardiomyoplasty. *Ann Thorac Surg* 56:1045–1053, 1993.
43. Akhmedov Sh, Krivoschekov E, Perkaskaya M, et al: Cardiomyoplasty in the treatment of heart failure patients. *Reblampa* 8:141S–144S, 1995.
44. Cohn JN: Structural basis for heart failure: Ventricular remodeling and its pharmacological inhibition. *Circulation* 91:2504–2507, 1995.
45. Packer M. Pathophysiology of chronic heart failure. *Lancet* 340:88–93, 1992.
46. Moreira LFP, Stolf NAG, Bocchi EA, et al: Clinical and left ventricular function outcomes up to five years after dynamic cardiomyoplasty. *J Thorac Cardiovasc Surg* 109:353–363, 1995.
47. Bocchi EA, Moreira LFP, Moraes AV, et al: Arrhythmias and sudden death after dynamic cardiomyoplasty. *Circulation* 90:II-107–II-111, 1994.
48. Huang SK, Messer JV, Denes P: Significance of ventricular tachycardia in idiopathic dilated cardiomyopathy. *Am J Cardiol* 51:507–512, 1993.

49. Borghetti-Maio SA, Romano BW, Bocchi EA, et al: Quality of life after cardiomyoplasty. *J Heart Lung Transpl* 13:271–275, 1994.
50. Bocchi EA, Guimarães GV, Moreira LFP, et al: Peak oxygen consumption and resting left ventricular ejection fraction changes after cardiomyoplasty at 6-month follow-up. *Circulation* 1995, in press.
51. Furnary AP, Chachques JC, Moreira LFP, et al: Long-term outcome, survival analysis and risk stratification of dynamic cardiomyoplasty. *J Thorac Cardiovasc Surg* 1995, in press.
52. Larsen L, Markham J, Haffajee CI: Sudden death in idiopathic dilated cardiomyopathy: Role of ventricular arrhythmias. *PACE* 16:1051–1059, 1993.
53. Moreira LFP, Seferian P Jr, Bocchi EA, et al: Survival improvement with dynamic cardiomyoplasty in patients with dilated cardiomyopathy. *Circulation* 84:III-296–III-302, 1991.
54. The SOLVD Investigators: Effect of enalapril on survival in patiients with reduced left ventricular ejection fractions and congestive heart failure. *N Engl J Med* 325:293–302, 1991.
55. Cohn JN, Johnson G, Ziesche S, et al. A comparison of enalapril with hydralazine–isosorbide dinitrate in the treatment of chronic congestive heart failure. *N Engl J Med* 325:303–310, 1991.
56. Morley D, Brozena SC: Assessing risk by hemodynamic profile in patients awaiting cardiac transplantation. *Am J Cardiol* 73:379–383, 1994.
57. Lucas CMHB, van der Veen FH, Chachques LC, et al: Long-term follow-up (12–35 weeks) after dynamic cardiomyoplasty. *J Am Coll Cardiol* 22:758–767, 1993.
58. Kratz JM, Johnson WS, Mukherjee R, et al: The relation between latissimus dorsi skeletal muscle structure and contractile function after cardiomyoplasty. *J Thorac Cardiovasc Surg* 107:868–878, 1994.
59. Kalil-Filho R, Bocchi EA, Weiss RG, et al: Magnetic resonance imaging evaluation of chronic changes in the latissimus dorsi cardiomyoplasty. *Circulation* 90:II-102–II-106, 1994.
60. Gealow K, Solien E, Bianco R, et al: Importance of adaptive stimulation of the latissimus dorsi muscle in cardiomyoplasty. *J Am Soc Artif Int Organs* 40:253–259, 1994.
61. Isoda S, Yano Y, Jin Y, et al: Influence of a delay on latissimus dorsi muscle flap blood flow. *Ann Thorac Surg* 59:632–638, 1995.
62. Fritzsche D, Krakor R, Asmussen G, et al: Anabolic steroids (Metenolone) improve performance and hemodynamic characteristics in cardiomyoplasty. *Ann Thorac Surg* 59:961–970, 1995.
63. Thakur RK, Chow LH, Guiraudon GM, et al: Latissimus dorsi dynamic cardiomyoplasty: Role of combined ICD implantation. *J Card Surg* 10:295–297, 1995.
64. Bolling SF, Deeb M, Brunsting LA, et al: Early outcome of mitral valve reconstruction in patients with end-stage cardiomyopathy. *J Thorac Cardiovasc Surg* 109:679–683, 1995.

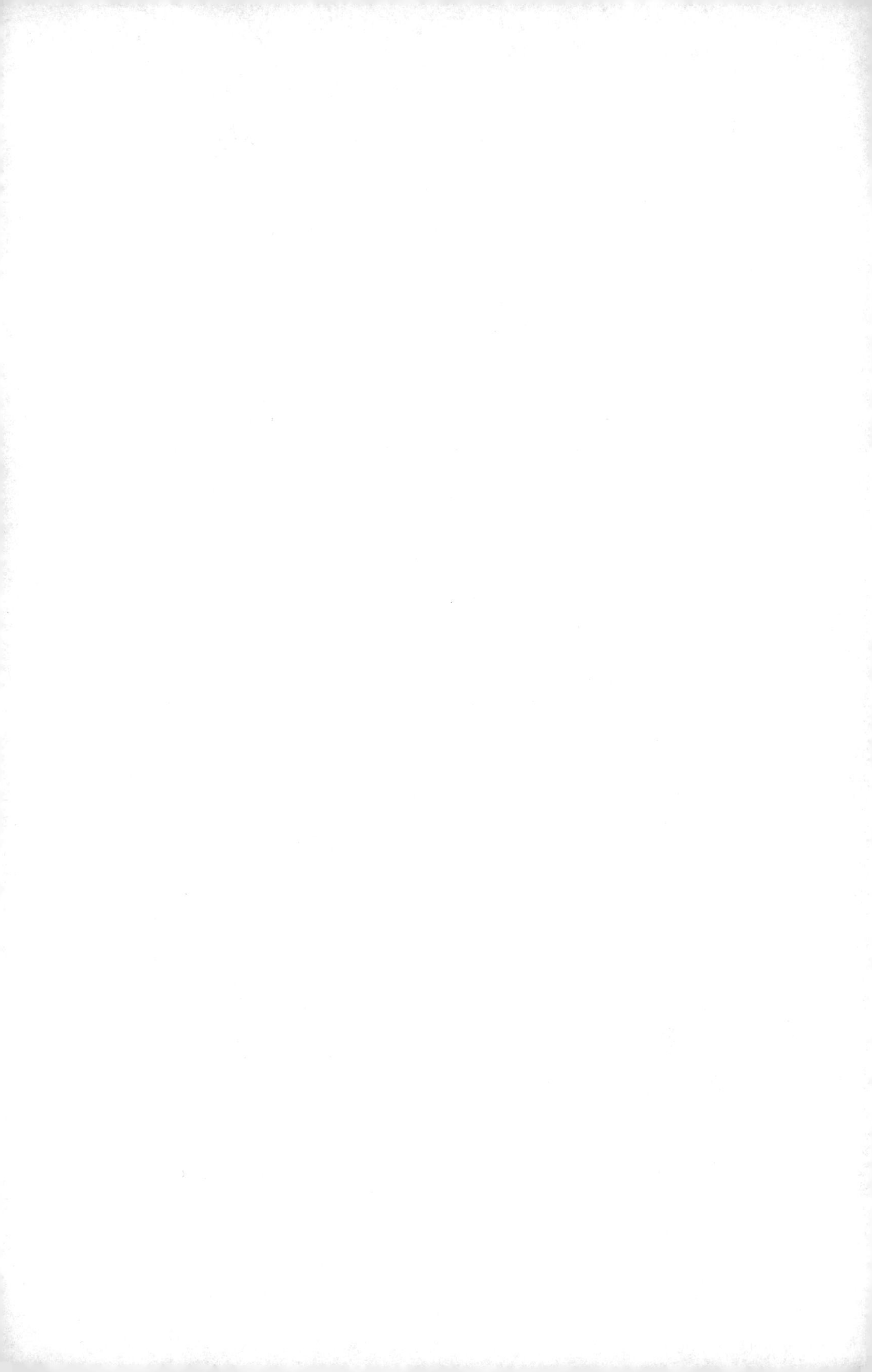

Index

A

B

L

M

N

O

P